Karen Hertz • Julie Santy-Tomlinson
Editors

Fragility Fracture Nursing

Holistic Care and Management of the Orthogeriatric Patient

Editors
Karen Hertz
Royal Stoke University Hospital
University Hospitals of North Midlands
Stoke-on-Trent
United Kingdom

Julie Santy-Tomlinson
Division of Nursing
Midwifery and Social Work
School of Health Sciences
University of Manchester
Manchester
United Kingdom

https://doi.org/10.1007/978-3-319-76681-2

Foreword

One of the biggest public health challenges we now face globally is the tsunami of hip and other fragility fractures, which is the consequence of rapidly ageing populations worldwide. In developed economies, this process has been under way for many years, and we have had the time to learn that there are two innovations that can help us cope with the challenge. They are (1) orthopaedic–geriatric co-management of the acute fracture episode and (2) secondary prevention, reliably delivered by a Fracture Liaison Service model.

One notable aspect of both these innovations is that their successful implementation is heavily dependent on the involvement of specially trained nurses. This is not only because the number of patients involved is so huge and there are simply not enough doctors available to deliver what is needed; it is also because skilled, highly educated nurses can collaboratively coordinate and deliver excellent care over the full 24-h period—with a significant impact on outcomes. This is even more true in those countries where population ageing is happening later and at a more hectic pace—particularly in emerging economies, but also many countries in Europe. Unfortunately, these tend to be countries in which the health services culture is inimical to autonomous action and decision-taking by nurses.

The nurse-education project which has produced this book, therefore, has twin goals:

1. To define the knowledge base and skill set that nurses need to be professionally competent to deliver the care that fragility fracture patients need
2. To assert the *appropriateness* of the delivery of such care by nurses with a fair degree of autonomy, albeit in the context of protocols that are developed and monitored in collaboration with the relevant medical specialists.

The process by which the book has been produced is itself a manifestation of this philosophy. The chapters were brainstormed in sessions containing, and led by, nurse leaders from 29 European countries, with minimal input from a handful of medical advisors. Meticulous preparation of these sessions by the editors ensured that the important issues were addressed and that the seminal studies that produced the relevant evidence for each issue were known and available to participants. This educational nurse meeting was hosted by Prof. Stefania Maggi and the European Interdisciplinary Council on Aging (EICA) in San Servolo Island, Venice Lagoon,

15/16 May 2017. The project was endorsed by the major international organisations concerned with osteoporosis and fragility fracture (EFORT, ESCEO, EUGMS, FFN, IAGG-ER, ICON and IOF).

We know that this is a work in progress that will have to be updated as more evidence accumulates. We also know that maximum benefit will be realised only when the material has been translated into many different languages and, in some respects, modified for different health care systems. We are confident that these things will happen, again, led by nurses.

We are very grateful to Springer for agreeing to make this English version available on the Internet for open access and to UCB for their unconditional financial support. This will speed up the roll-out process considerably. We are sure that this open access educational nursing book will greatly contribute to the growth of nursing community all over the world in the field of osteoporosis and fragility fractures.

David Marsh
University College London
London, UK

Fragility Fracture Network
Zurich, Switzerland

Paolo Falaschi
Fragility Fracture Network
Zurich, Switzerland

Sapienza University of Rome
Roma, Italy

Preface

Patients with fragility fractures are the most common orthopaedic trauma inpatients, found in great numbers in every acute hospital in every country. Their care is provided in hospital units as well as pre-hospital care settings, emergency departments, outpatient clinics, rehabilitation units and community settings. Despite their high numbers and presence in a wide range of settings, nurses have rarely received formal education in the care and management of this vulnerable group of patients and the centrality of the nursing role is not well recognised in the literature. The aim of this book (as well as the associated educational programme) is to ensure that this is resolved.

Patients who have sustained a fragility fracture are usually elderly and often frail. Although many may have suffered a relatively minor fracture that can be treated as an outpatient, such injuries are warning signs of a fracture that is the result of fragile bone caused by osteoporosis, which requires treatment to prevent further fractures. Those patients requiring hospitalisation often have a hip fracture, a significant injury that nearly always requires major orthopaedic surgery and places significant physiological and psychological stress on the patient, potentially leading to significant reduction in function and mobility, loss of independence, complications and death.

There are several different models of care, not only nationally but internationally, and not everyone gets the same care or the care they deserve. Hospitalisation may result in admission to a general orthopaedic trauma unit, but increasingly health services are recognising the unique needs of this group of frail and vulnerable patients and are developing 'enhanced care' units, often known as orthogeriatric units or hip fracture wards/units, where there is access to specialist medical and nursing care that includes geriatricians and other members of a multidisciplinary team with advanced skills in caring for patients with highly complex needs following a fracture. Patients are often frail and have multiple co-morbidities. Their preparation and recovery from surgery requires optimisation so that these factors are not only considered but actively managed. Patients whose care and management is not optimised have very poor outcomes in terms of regaining functional abilities and experience prolonged pain and complications that can, ultimately, lead to death.

Nurses caring for this group of hospital patients require provision of evidence-based, multidisciplinary care that brings together the skills and knowledge of acute orthopaedic care, acute geriatric care, rehabilitation, and palliative care. This requires both advanced knowledge and enhanced skills. However, this is not the complete picture: patients with fragility fractures also need skilled and professional care in community and outpatient settings with a particular focus on bone health and fracture prevention. What is special about nurses and nursing is that they spend more time than any other member of the team with patients, in or outside the hospital, and often provide care over the full 24-h period. They have a different skill set from other members of the multidisciplinary team and can work at different levels from novice through to expert [1]. At all of these levels, nurses perceive and understand patients' care needs holistically and are able to provide high-quality care.

This book has been written by a group of expert nurses, each with skills and knowledge in specific aspects of fragility fracture care. The group were brought together for the first time in May 2017, on the Island of San Servolo, Venice Lagoon, Italy, as part of a project aimed at designing an education programme with the specific goal of improving the care of fragility fracture patients across Europe. At that meeting a 'big conversation' took place about what nurses need to know in order to provide excellent nursing care. Even in the short time since that meeting, the project's reach has begun to extend well beyond Europe and the venture has become known as the 'San Servolo Project'.

Each contributor has a different background, offering the opportunity for the book to truly bring together a depth of experience of multidisciplinary practice and to acknowledge the need for practice development across a world where local practice varies according to social, cultural and political influences. For example, in some countries there are no geriatricians to act as clinical leaders for fragility fracture care and local nursing practice has developed accordingly. Despite the differences in local practice, what we noticed was consistent when we discussed nursing and fragility fracture care for the first time in San Servolo was the prominence of the team approach and multi/interdisciplinary working in those conversations, a prominence that is now reflected in this book. There is strength in a team that is much more than the sum of its parts. That team also includes the patient and his/her family, friends and informal caregivers. This reflects the ethos of the Fragility Fracture Network (FFN http://fragilityfracturenetwork.org/), an organisation aimed at optimising globally '...the multidisciplinary management of the patient with a fragility fracture, including secondary prevention', with nurses participating as equals, offering complementary knowledge and skills to the other members of the team.

The wealth of fragility fracture/orthogeriatric knowledge presented in this book is accessible to all nurses who care for these patients in any setting and, we hope, will be available to the next generation of nurses who want to practise in this challenging field and continue to improve care. This knowledge comes from the evidence base, as well as the diverse and extensive experience of the contributors. The chapters will provide the reader with a wealth of information that they can apply to their practices, but their learning should not finish at the end of the book. It should go on to be continuous: through the suggestions for further study and self-assessment at the end of each chapter and beyond. The chapters will help nurses to develop their orthogeriatric knowledge and skills so that they can provide care that reflects it them. This process will involve deepening their knowledge about the causes of fragility fracture—specifically bone fragility due to osteoporosis and falls. It also involves understanding the importance of a well-led systematic approach to bone health, falls and fracture prevention.

Comprehensive assessment of the older person with a fragility fracture, especially hip fracture, is central to effective, evidence-based care in the emergency, perioperative and recovery periods, and an understanding of frailty and sarcopenia underpins all of this. Many aspects of care are discussed, but pain management, complication prevention, remobilisation, nutrition, hydration, wound management and pressure ulcer prevention are singled out for specific attention here because they are so central to improving patient outcomes and, so, are intertwined with nursing. Delirium and other cognitive impairments such as dementia are, like depression, major insults to the recovery and rehabilitation of patients following fragility fracture and surgery and need to be carefully managed. Nurses also need to be aware that, in some cases, hip fracture may be the beginning of the final phase of a person's life and that sensitive palliative care, with effective symptom control and emotional and psychological support for patients and their families may also been needed. Nurses are well placed to do all of this with the collaboration of the patient and his/her family.

Sharing knowledge and skills nationally and internationally through local, national and global organisations such as local and national nursing groups, the Fragility Fracture Network (FFN) and the International Collaboration of Orthopaedic Nurses (ICON) is an integral part of the development of nursing practice.

This is a 'sister' book to *Orthogeriatrics* edited by Falaschi and Marsh [2]. Numerous medical organisations with members specialising in bone health and fragility fracture have, to date, supported the San Servolo Project including the European Interdisciplinary Council on Aging (EICA) and has been endorsed by the major international organisations concerned with osteoporosis and fragility fracture (EFORT, ESCEO, EUGMS, FFN, IAGG-ER, ICON and IOF). Recently, this culminated in an unrestricted educational grant from our industry partner, UCB, enabling the book to be published online as an open access eBook so that the education it offers is freely available to all nurses across the globe, no matter what their location or income. This support has been freely offered because every individual and organisation believes in the power of nursing to make the care of patients with fragility fractures the very best it can be so that their suffering can be much less and their outcomes much better.

Stoke-on-Trent, UK — Karen Hertz
Manchester, UK — Julie Santy-Tomlinson

References

1. Benner PE (1984) From novice to expert: excellence and power in clinical nursing practice. Addison-Wesley, Menlo Park
2. Falaschi P, Marsh D (eds) (2017) Orthogeriatrics. Springer, Cham

Acknowledgment

Open access publication has been possible through an unconditioned educational grant from UCB

Contents

About the Editors

Karen Hertz is is a registered nurse with extensive experience of clinical practice in a wide range of acute hospital settings with a focus on orthopaedic/trauma and orthogeriatric nursing as well as all aspects of adult nursing. She has developed a clinical career in the role of Advanced Nurse Practitioner in which she provides patient focused care, using advanced assessments skills and nurse prescribing privileges to provide autonomous clinical practice for patients within a trauma unit in a large University Hospital. She has a track record of national and international networking that includes membership of various boards and committees relevant to her practice and has co-authored several book chapters.

Dr. Julie Santy-Tomlinson is a registered nurse with clinical interests in orthopaedics and trauma, wound management, tissue viability and nursing care of the older adult. She has worked in nursing education in the UK for over 20 years and currently works at the University of Manchester as a Senior Lecturer where she teaches a broad spectrum of nursing topics. She is also Editor in Chief of the *International Journal of Orthopaedic and Trauma Nursing* and has authored, co-authored and co-edited numerous journal papers, clinical guidelines, books and book chapters.

Abbreviations

AADLs	Advanced activities of daily living
ABCDE	Airway, breathing, circulation, disability, exposure
ADLs	Activities of daily living
APIE	Assessment, planning, implementation and evaluation
BADLs	Basic activities of daily living
BMD	Bone mineral density
BMI	Body mass index
BOA	British Orthopaedic Association
BP	Blood pressure
CGA	Comprehensive Geriatric Assessment
DAI	Deficit Accumulation Index
DVT	Deep vein thrombosis
DXA	Dual-energy X-ray absorptiometry
ED	Emergency Department
EWGSOP	European Working Group on Sarcopenia in Older People
FFN	Fragility Fracture Network
FLS	Fracture Liaison Service
HAI	Hospital acquired infection
IAD	Incontinence-associated dermatitis
IADLs	Instrumental or intermediate activities of daily living
ICP	Integrated care pathway
ICN	International Council of Nurses
IOF	International Osteoporosis Foundation
ITD	Intertriginous dermatitis
MARS	Medical adhesive-related skin injury
MASD	Moisture-associated skin damage
MDT	Multidisciplinary team
NOF	National Osteoporosis Federation
NOS	National Osteoporosis Society
ONJ	Osteonecrosis of the jaw
PE	Pulmonary embolism
PFP	Physical Frailty Phenotype
QoL	Quality of life
RDA	Recommended daily dietary allowance

SD	Standard deviations
SERM	Selective Estrogen Receptor Modulator
SOF	Study of Osteoporotic Fractures
UTI	Urinary tract infection
VFA	Vertebral Fracture Assessment
VTE	Venous thromboembolism
WHO	World Health Organization

Contributors

Silvia Barberi Azienda Ospedaliera San Giovanni Addolorata, Rome, Italy

Louise Brent National Office of Clinical Audit, Dublin, Ireland

Panagiota Copanitsanou Department of Orthopaedics and Traumatology, General Hospital of Piraeus "Tzaneio", Piraeus, Greece

National and Kapodistrian University of Athens, Athens, Greece

Jason Cross POPS Team (Proactive care of the Older Person undergoing Surgery), Guys and St Thomas' NHS Foundation Trust, London, UK

Karen Hertz University Hospital of North Midlands, Stoke-on-Trent, UK

Ami Hommel Department of Orthopaedics, Skane University Hospital, Malmö, Sweden

Department of Care Science, Malmö University, Malmö, Sweden

Charlotte Myhre Jensen Department of Orthopaedic Surgery and Traumatology, Odense University Hospital, Odense, Denmark

Magdalena Kamińska Department of Primary Health Care, Faculty of Health Sciences, Pomeranian Medical University, Szczecin, Poland

Andréa Marques Serviço de Reumatologia, Consulta Externa 7° piso, Centro Hospitalar e Universitário de Coimbra, Coimbra, Portugal

Oliver Mauthner Felix Platter, Spital, University of Basel, Basel, Switzerland

Lucia Mielli Azienda Sanitaria Unica Regionale (ASUR), Distretto Sanitario di S. Benedetto del Tronto, Marche, Italy

Carmen Queirós Centro Hospitalar do Porto, Escola Superior de Enfermagem do Porto, Porto, Portugal

Patrick Roigk Abteilung für Geriatrie und Klinik für Geriatrische Rehabilitation/ Department of Clinical Gerontology and Rehabilitation, Robert-Bosch-Krankenhaus/Robert-Bosch-Hospital, Stuttgart, Germany

Julie Santy-Tomlinson School of Health Sciences, University of Manchester, Manchester, UK

Robyn Speerin Musculoskeletal Network, NSW Agency for Clinical Innovation, Chatswood, NSW, Australia

Lina Spirgienė Department of Nursing and Care, Medical Academy, Faculty of Nursing, Lithuanian University of Health Sciences, Kaunas, Lithuania

Hospital of Lithuanian University of Health Sciences, Kaunas, Lithuania

Ana Cruz Tochon-Laruaz Fracture Liaison Service, Geneva University Hospitals, Genève, Switzerland

Marsha van Oostwaard Osteoporosis—Endocrinology, Màxima Medisch Centrum, Veldhoven, The Netherlands

Osteoporosis and the Nature of Fragility Fracture: An Overview

1

Marsha van Oostwaard

The main consequence of osteoporosis is that it is a condition in which bone mass is depleted and bone structure is destroyed to the degree that bone becomes fragile and prone to fractures. For affected patients, these 'fragility fractures' are associated with substantial pain and suffering, disability and even death, along with substantial costs to society. The problems created by fragility fractures and osteoporosis are multifactorial in origin and are, therefore, a multidisciplinary problem. A first fragility fracture is often the early sign of osteoporosis, and 'secondary' prevention of fragility fractures is focused on the prevention of further fractures once an initial fracture has occurred. Nurses play a key role in education and guidance of patients with osteoporosis. This chapter will provide an overview of how osteoporosis and fragility fractures are linked, with a focus on fracture prevention.

1.1 Learning Outcomes

At the end of the chapter, and following further study, the nurse will be able to:

- Explain the basics of bone biology and its relationship to osteoporosis and fragility fractures.
- Describe the most common fragility fractures and their impact on individuals.
- Undertake fracture risk assessment and recognise and modify the fixed and modifiable risk factors using the FRAX© calculation tool.

M. van Oostwaard
Màxima Medisch Centrum, Veldhoven, Netherlands
e-mail: M.vanOostwaard@mmc.nl

K. Hertz, J. Santy-Tomlinson (eds.), *Fragility Fracture Nursing*, Perspectives in Nursing Management and Care for Older Adults, https://doi.org/10.1007/978-3-319-76681-2_1

- Educate communities and individuals about osteoporosis diagnosis and treatment and advise on lifestyle.
- Outline the goals and benefits of osteoporosis treatment, and support individuals during treatment.

1.2 Bone Biology

The human skeleton gives structure to the body and protects organs, makes motion and mobility possible by attachment to muscles via tendons and ligaments, stores and releases minerals and, in the bone marrow, manufactures blood cells. About 80% of the skeleton is cortical (or compact) bone that forms the outer structure of the shafts of long bones. Trabecular bone (20%) is mainly present in the ends of long bones and in the centre of the vertebrae and ribs. Bone undergoes a lifelong process of replacement; mature bone is replaced with new. This regulated process of 'bone turnover' maintains a balance between bone resorption and formation to maintain skeletal integrity [1] and results in replacement of 5–10% of the skeleton each year and the total skeleton every decade [2].

Remodelling involves three types of cells; osteoblasts (bone builders), osteoclasts (bone eaters) and osteocytes, and is a continuous interaction between hormones, minerals and bone cells that is influenced by; (1) changes in calcium levels in the blood, (2) pressure/strain on the bones caused by gravity and the action of muscles and (3) hormones (oestrogen, testosterone and growth hormone).

In youth, bone formation exceeds resorption, so bone mass and strength increase. Peak bone mass is achieved between the ages of 20 and 25 years [3]. At 30–40 years, bone mass gradually decreases as bone resorption exceeds bone formation. It is estimated that, by the age of 80, total bone mass is ±50% of its peak [4]. When the balance tips towards excessive resorption, bones weaken (osteopenia) and, over time, can become brittle and at risk of fracture (osteoporosis) [5].

1.3 Osteoporosis

Osteoporosis is a common chronic systemic skeletal disease that is 'characterised by low bone mass and microarchitectural deterioration of bone tissue, with a consequent increase in bone fragility and susceptibility to fracture' [6] (see Fig. 1.1). It is a devastating disease that can lead to pain, severe disability and premature death from fracture. As bones become more porous and fragile, the more the risk of fracture is increased. Patients are often unaware they are at risk of or have osteoporosis because bone loss occurs silently and progressively without signs or symptoms until fractures occur.

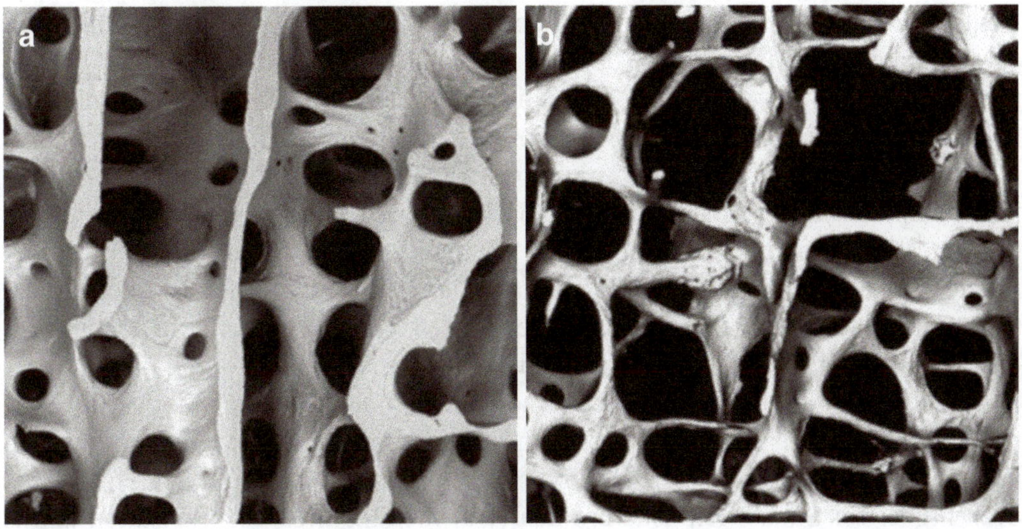

Fig. 1.1 Microscopic structure of normal and osteoporotic bone (**a**) Normal bone and (**b**) Osteoporotic bone (©Alan Boyde 2018 with permission)

1.4 Epidemiology

Osteoporosis is a global problem, but the size of the problem is unclear because of the variability in assessment and awareness. In Europe, India, Japan and the USA, there are an estimated 125 million people suffering from osteoporosis. Globally, one in three women and one in five men will experience a fragility fracture resulting in a hospital visit every 3 s. In 2010, in the EU alone, 22 million women and 5.5 million men were estimated to have osteoporosis, resulting in 3.5 million new fragility fractures, comprising 610,000 hip fractures, 520,000 vertebral fractures, 560,000 forearm fractures and 1,800,000 other fractures. The economic burden was estimated at €37 billion and is still rising [7]. After hip fracture, for example, 40% of patients cannot walk independently, 80% cannot perform basic activities such as shopping independently, and 10–20% need permanent residential care [8]. The number of people living with osteoporosis in all global regions will increase dramatically in the coming decades due to ageing populations and lifestyle changes. The costs are expected to increase by 25% by 2025.

1.5 Fragility Fracture and Osteoporosis

'Fragility fractures occur as a result of "low energy trauma", often from a fall from standing height or less, that would not normally result in a fracture' [9] and they are a major public health problem; one occurs globally every 3 s, with high human and socio-economic impact, morbidity, mortality and costs. For individuals, fractures frequently result in loss of autonomy, deterioration in quality of life and need for care. A fragility fracture may be defined as a pathological fracture that results from minimal trauma (e.g. a fall from a standing height) or no identifiable trauma at all [8]. The fracture is both a sign and a symptom of osteoporosis.

Typical fractures in patients with osteoporosis include vertebral (spine), proximal femur (hip), distal forearm (wrist) and proximal humerus [10]. Wrist fractures are the third most common type of osteoporotic fractures, accounting for up to 18% of all fractures among the elderly [11], and their impact on quality of life due to complications and impaired function is often underestimated. These distal forearm fractures are often 'the first' fragility fracture, followed by a subsequent hip or vertebral fracture.

Hip fractures are the most serious fractures. Although a woman's risk of dying from a hip fracture is high, and exceeds the lifetime risk of death from breast cancer, uterine cancer and ovarian cancer combined, the mortality risk after a hip fracture is even higher for a man. Hip fracture nearly always requires hospitalisation and is fatal in almost a quarter of all cases. For those who survive, most do not regain their pre-injury level of function, and 30% experience loss of independence. Dependency is greatly feared by patients and is costly to their family and to society [12]. If a first fragility fracture is recognised and osteoporosis treated, the risk of a future fracture can be reduced by approximately 50%, preventing the downward spiral in health and quality of life that often follows hip fracture.

Vertebral fractures are the most common manifestation of osteoporosis and are usually diagnosed when a patient presents with back pain and has a spinal X-ray that shows vertebral body fracture. Patients may have spinal fractures but never be aware of them; only 25% are clinically diagnosed as they are often asymptomatic or mildly symptomatic. Hence, although they are common, the majority do not come to attention at the time they occur, so vertebral fractures in older adults are associated with an increased mortality, often due to frailty (Chap. 2) [13]. Recognised vertebral fractures are usually treated non-surgically with a brief period of bed rest, pain medication, bracing and physiotherapy. Approximately 40% of patients develop chronic disabling pain and/or spinal deformity (kyphosis) resulting in reduced pulmonary function associated with increased risk of mortality. Vertebral fractures increase the risk of sustaining future fractures fivefold, so it is important to identify them and start treatment. If a vertebral fracture occurs when patients are already being treated for osteoporosis, therapy requires evaluation and adjustment.

It is important to identify patients with increased fracture risk. Nurses can play a key role in assessing risk factors while obtaining a medical history when patients attend for hospital treatment following a fracture. Investing in fracture risk assessment and education for risk reduction is an important potential intervention. Following assessment of risk factors and lifestyle change education, measures can be taken to impact on modifiable risk factors and meet the individual's need for information and education.

1.5.1 Risk Factors

Risk factors for osteoporosis and fracture can be divided into two categories. Fixed risk factors (listed in Box 1.1) cannot be modified but help to identify patients with high fracture risk [14].

Box 1.1: Fixed Risk Factors for Osteoporosis [15]

Age: from 50 years, fracture risk increases, with doubling of risk for every decade thereafter because bone mineral density decreases and other risk factors such as falling or comorbidities increase.

Female gender: women are more at risk of developing osteoporosis due to menopausal decrease in oestrogen. Women have a lower peak bone mass than men.

Family history of osteoporosis: having a parent with a hip fracture at any time in their lives is associated with an increased risk of fracture (independent of bone mineral density).

Previous fracture: doubles the risk of a second fracture in both men and women.

Ethnicity: Caucasian and Asian people have a higher incidence of osteoporosis and fractures of the hip and spine.

Menopause: osteoclasts are more active, and bone loss increases due to decrease in oestrogen levels following menopause or oophorectomy.

Long-term glucocorticoid therapy: increases bone loss and impairs bone formation and calcium absorption and muscle weakness can increase the risk of falling.

Rheumatoid arthritis: inflammatory cytokines and impaired mobility increase bone loss.

Primary/secondary hypogonadism in men: rapidly increases bone loss due to normal ageing or following orchidectomy or androgen deprivation therapy.

Secondary risk factors: disorders and medications that make the bone more fragile and/or effect balance (increasing risk of falling). Also including immobility, inflammatory bowel diseases, eating disorders and endocrine disorders.

Most modifiable risk factors (listed in Box 1.2) directly impact on bone biology and result in a decrease in bone mineral density, but can also increase the risk of fracture independently of their effect on bone itself. Nurses can educate and guide patients towards healthier lifestyles to reduce these risk factors.

Box 1.2: Modifiable Risk Factors for Osteoporosis [14]

Alcohol: Excessive alcohol consumption (>2 U daily) increases the risk of a fracture by 40% due to direct adverse effects on osteoblasts and parathyroid hormone levels (regulates calcium metabolism); associated with poor nutritional status (calcium, protein and vitamin D deficiency) [15].

Smoking: The exact mechanism is unknown, but increased fracture risk is reported when there is a history of cigarette smoking [16].

Low body mass index (BMI): Regardless of age, sex and weight loss, BMI <20 kg/m^2 is associated with a twofold increased risk of fracture compared to people with a BMI of 25 kg/m^2.

Poor nutrition: Inadequate intake of calcium, vitamin D or both will influence calcium-regulating hormones; deficiency of either calcium or vitamin D will result in impaired calcium absorption and lower concentration of circulating calcium; parathyroid hormone (PTH) secretion is stimulated, increasing PTH levels and leading to an increase in bone remodelling, significant loss of bone and increased risk of fracture.

Vitamin D deficiency: Vitamin D plays an essential role in calcium absorption; it is made in the skin when exposed to the sun's ultraviolet rays (10–15 min a day is usually sufficient); food sources (see Chap. 8) or supplemental sources of vitamin D are beneficial [17].

Eating disorders: Due to poor nutrition and vitamin D deficiency and obtaining a lower peak bone mass in early adulthood.

Oestrogen deficiency: Accelerates bone loss and reduces the build-up of bone mass; related to both hormone imbalance (e.g. menopause) and nutritional factors.

Insufficient exercise: Due to sedentary lifestyle (e.g. women who sit down for > 9 h/day are 50% more likely to fracture a hip than those who sit for <6 h/day); bone remodelling is regulated by mechanical load; load-bearing physical activity and muscle activity; placing tension and torsion on bone is detected by osteocytes.

Low dietary calcium intake: (See Chap. 8.)

Frequent falls: Factors that increase risk of falling (see Chap. 3).

Low bone mineral density (BMD), one of the most important indicators of fracture risk, is both a fixed and modifiable risk factor determined by a wide range of factors, including family history, age and lifestyle. Prevention of osteoporosis starts in youth by gaining a sufficient peak bone mass; it is estimated that a 10% increase in the peak bone mass of children reduces the risk of an osteoporotic fracture during adulthood by 50%. Children should be encouraged to exercise and play outside and should be given vitamin D supplements (within national guidelines) alongside a healthy diet with sufficient calcium intake. When an individual is diagnosed with osteoporosis, prevention is no longer about gaining a higher bone mass but preventing fractures. Treatment of osteoporosis consists of prescription of specific anti-osteoporosis medication and calcium and vitamin D supplements in combination with healthy lifestyles.

Nurses can play a key role in fracture prevention by identifying patients at risk, educating patients about healthy diet, recommending adequate uptake of vitamin D, encouraging regular weight-bearing activity and supporting smoking cessation and alcohol consumption reduction.

Diagnosis and treatment of osteoporosis include; (1) case finding, (2) risk evaluation, (3) differential diagnosis of secondary osteoporosis, (4) therapy/treatment and (5) follow-up.

1.5.2 Diagnosis

All nurses who provide care to older people and those who have already sustained a fragility fracture should be aware of the possibility of their patients having osteoporosis and an increased risk of a next fracture (Table 1.1). They must know how to assess and modify the risk factors, why and how osteoporosis is diagnosed and how to ensure that proper referrals are made to other members of the multidisciplinary team.

Patients who have been diagnosed with this chronic condition need support in developing coping strategies. Most newly diagnosed patients are afraid of sustaining another fracture and feel vulnerable, sometimes leading to a paralysing fear of falling. Patients with advanced osteoporosis often experience decreased ability to perform activities of daily living and suffer from chronic back pain along with depression, loss of self-esteem, disability and increasing physical dependence. Nurses can advocate and educate by helping patients to maintain function and improve quality of life [18] and can refer patients to national osteoporosis associations for further information and support.

1.5.3 Case Finding

Case finding involves opportunistically identifying patients with osteoporosis when they present with a first fracture, using the fracture (a risk factor itself) as the starting point. This is the first step towards identifying those patients most urgently in need of fracture prevention through one of two approaches:

- *Primary prevention*: preventing the first fracture by identifying patient risk factors and starting treatment; often in primary healthcare settings where there may be a lack of structured or organised programmes.
- *Secondary prevention*: preventing a second fracture after the first; assessment and treatment is performed in hospitals using structured programmes such as fracture liaison services (FLS) (Chap. 3) and often initiated in the emergency department (ED).

1.5.4 Risk Evaluation

Bone mineral density (BMD) is a measure of bone strength estimated by dual-energy X-ray absorptiometry (DXA). Low BMD is the strongest risk factor for fracture. Clinical diagnosis of osteoporosis is based on BMD measurements and the presence of fractures [19]; BMD is transformed into a T-score, which reflects the number of standard deviations (SD) above or below the mean in healthy young adults. The thresholds for each bone category are shown in Table 1.1.

The DXA scan gives an *estimation* of bone strength by measuring the BMD in g/ cm^2 in an area of the lumbar spine (L1–4), the proximal femur and hip with little or no radiation exposure (20 μSv). Every decrease of 1 SD increases the risk of a fracture approximately twofold [20]. The cortical and trabecular structures of the bone are also associated with fragility fractures, highlighting that fracture risk is not only about BMD but must be approached as multifactorial. DXA measurements can be negatively influenced by failing to position the patient properly, recent ingestion of barium for abdominal investigation, presence of vertebral fractures in the L1–4 region, hip prostheses, degenerative skeletal problems and severe arterial calcifications.

As vertebral fractures are often asymptomatic, it is essential to identify them during assessment. Most DXA scanners can also perform an additional investigation of the spine at the same time, Vertebral Fracture Assessment (VFA). The results are methodically assessed according to the Genant classification (Table 1.2). The presence of a vertebral fracture is always a sign of impaired bone strength, a predictor of a next fracture and an indication for treatment. Vertebral fractures can also be identified by X-ray when VFA is inconclusive or not available.

Another way to estimate the risk of fracture is by using the FRAX© calculation tool, a validated web-based risk assessment tool in the form of a questionnaire (12 questions) that calculates the 10-year risk of fracture based on individual risk factors with or without a known BMD. FRAX© is integrated into many national guidelines, is available in multiple languages, is easy and quick to use and is available to any healthcare professional through a website and mobile applications. It can assist in targeting patients needing intervention and can be used by all [21].

Table 1.1 WHO criteria for clinical diagnosis of osteoporosis [19]

BMD T-score	Diagnosis
T-score ≥ −1 SD	Normal
−1 > T-score > −2.5 SD	Low bone mass/osteopenia
T-score ≤ −2.5 SD	Osteoporosis
T-score ≤ −2.5 SD with existing fracture	Severe osteoporosis

Table 1.2 Genant classification

Normal vertebra	Grade 0		
Mild fracture	Grade 1	−20–25%	Wedge, biconcave or crush
Moderate fracture	Grade 2	−25–40%	Wedge, biconcave or crush
Severe fracture	Grade 3	≥−40%	Wedge, biconcave or crush

1.5.5 Differential Diagnosis of Secondary Osteoporosis

Approximately 30% of women and 50% of men with osteoporosis have secondary osteoporosis that may be known or hidden and is caused by specific clinical conditions (Box 1.3). Treating the cause can decrease fracture risk and avoid unnecessary treatment [22], so every patient with a fragility fracture and a low BMD should have a baseline blood test for bone and mineral metabolism (calcium, phosphate, alkaline phosphatase, 25-hydroxyvitamin D, parathyroid hormone), liver and kidney function, full blood count and thyroid-stimulating hormone.

Box 1.3: Examples of Disorders Associated with Secondary Osteoporosis

- Diabetes mellitus
- Cushing's syndrome
- Hyperparathyroidism
- Hyperthyroidism
- Premature menopause
- Hypogonadism
- Celiac disease
- Inflammatory bowel disease
- Liver cirrhosis
- Rheumatoid arthritis
- Ankylosing spondylitis
- Systemic lupus erythematosus
- Anorexia nervosa

1.5.6 Treatment

Many patients are unaware they have osteoporosis until after their first fracture, but even after a fracture, it often goes untreated. This international 'treatment gap' means fewer than 20% of those who sustain a fragility fracture receive therapies to reduce the risk of fracture within the year following the fracture [23]. Treatment of osteoporosis is a combination of medication, lifestyle choices, adequate intake of calcium and vitamin D and prevention of falls.

The goal of osteoporosis medication is to *prevent fractures* (not to increase the DXA numbers). Fracture risk can be reduced by approximately 50% with optimal treatment of osteoporosis that consists of:

- Specific anti-osteoporosis medication (agreed through shared decision-making)
- Adequate intake of calcium and vitamin D (dietary or supplements)
- Attention to lifestyle factors (hand in hand with prescribed drug treatment)
- Fall prevention (when relevant)
- Follow-up (plan is known by the patient).

1.5.6.1 Medication to Reduce Fracture Risk

There are various medications used to treat osteoporosis, all having different entry points, but they all have the same goal: preventing fractures. The most common approved treatments will be considered here including:

- Bisphosphonates (alendronate, ibandronate, risedronate and zoledronic acid) (oral or intravenous)
- 'Selective oestrogen receptor modulators' (SERM) (raloxifene, bazedoxifene; oestrogen 'agonist/antagonist' drugs that act like oestrogen in bone but in the uterus and breast tissue act like an oestrogen blocker)
- Parathyroid hormone (teriparatide): stimulates (new) bone formation, resulting in increased BMD (daily subcutaneously injection)
- Monoclonal antibody (denosumab): reduces bone turnover by inhibiting the maturation of osteoclasts (subcutaneously every 6 months).

While the development of new treatments is ongoing, the most commonly prescribed are bisphosphonates which attach to bone tissue and reduce bone turnover by suppressing the activity of osteoclasts, often referred to as 'anti-resorption' therapy. The drug must be taken regularly for a minimum of 5 years initially and is combined with calcium and vitamin D supplements. Oral bisphosphonates are poorly absorbed (only approximately 1% of each dose), even with total compliance and proper administration. When administered orally, bisphosphonates must be taken according to the following instructions:

- In the morning, on an empty stomach
- At least 30 min before any food or drink
- Swallowed whole with a large glass of tap water
- The patient must remain upright for at least 30 min
- Any calcium-containing supplements must be delayed for 3–4 h.

Proper follow-up improves adherence and compliance with treatment and facilitates monitoring of the treatment goal - fracture prevention. At the start of treatment, patients must be aware of the duration, the goal and benefits, for how long the medication must be taken and from whom to seek support when problems such as side effects occur. Many patients fail to persist with their treatment, and many others experience a suboptimal response due to unintentional poor compliance or impaired absorption. Approximately 50% of all patients who start treatment stop within the first year [24]. It is important to check regularly that patients are following the instructions and are continuing to take their treatment properly. Despite the wishes of most patients to measure the effect of the treatment short term, it is not recommended to make periodic measurements of BMD by DXA because BMD changes as a result of osteoporosis treatment occur slowly and the magnitude of measurement error with DXA is similar to the short-term change in response to treatment. An alternative approach is to measure biochemical markers of bone turnover in blood or urine samples. These show large and rapid changes in response to osteoporosis treatment, allowing detection of a significant treatment response within a few months.

Another factor in poor compliance is fear of side effects. In oral treatments, gastrointestinal complaints are a common reason for patients to stop the treatment without talking to their health practitioner. It is important that patients report side effects so that further treatment options can be discussed. A rare, but feared, side effect is osteonecrosis of the jaw (ONJ); the risk can be reduced by good oral hygiene and regular dental care.

All patients will have an individual treatment plan through life depending on the significance of their fracture risk, the type of medication and lifestyle changes. The duration of the different therapies varies, and there is no uniform recommendation that applies to all patients. After a period of treatment, re-evaluation of the risk should be performed, consisting of DXA, VFA (or X-ray of the spine) and fracture risk assessment. Treatment of osteoporosis is sometimes difficult for patients to understand, meaning that treatment plans sometimes fail. Patients need to know from diagnosis that osteoporosis is a chronic condition but that treatment duration is limited (bisphosphonates treatment is 3–5 years). Good understanding of diagnosis and fracture risk is important because patients can then make informed choices regarding treatment and lifestyle changes. Adherence and compliance are often low due to lack of knowledge, lack of guidance, invalid values and beliefs regarding therapies, side effects and the fact that patients do not 'feel' the benefits of the treatment, i.e. not having a fracture.

Nurses play a key role in improving compliance and adherence through specific nursing interventions including:

- Education about the treatment goal and benefits
- Education about the prescribed drug regimen and recognising significant adverse reactions
- Instructing the patient to report side effects
- Advising patients on how to properly administer the medication
- Assessing and supporting compliance and adherence
- Informing and recording for how long patients have to take their medication
- Scheduling fracture risk re-evaluation
- Advising on lifestyle modification regarding diet and exercise
- Advising on good oral hygiene and regular dental care
- Advising on prevention of falls (see Chaps. 2 and 3)
- Referring patients to national osteoporosis associations for support.

1.5.7 Suggested Further Study

To effectively provide care to patients with or at risk of fragility factures, it is essential that nurses have extensive and up-to-date knowledge of osteoporosis, its prevention and management. Individual further study should be conducted using the following:

- Talk to patients and their families about the impact of sustaining a fragility fracture due to osteoporosis. Reflect on these conversations, and search for evidence-based literature about improving care and outcomes.
- Expand knowledge by taking an online course, and use this to assess knowledge and performance anually.

- Read and make notes from books, articles and national or international guidelines on osteoporosis and fracture prevention. The following are examples, but many other options exist.

Online Courses

https://nos.org.uk/for-health-professionals/professional-development/e-learning-and-training/ — an interactive training course enabling any clinician to improve their knowledge and ability to deliver excellent healthcare to people with, or at risk of, osteoporosis and fragility fractures

https://www.cme.nof.org/BoneSource™ - NOF's professional programme, promotes excellence in clinical care for all healthcare professionals involved in the prevention, diagnosis and treatment of osteoporosis

Example Websites

www.capturethefracture.org/
www.iofbonehealth.org
www.nos.org.uk
www.nof.org

Suggested Reading

Curtis, E.M. Moon, R.J. Harvey, N.C. Cooper, C. (2017) The impact of fragility fracture and approaches to osteoporosis risk assessment worldwide. Bone. 104:29-38, 7-17 https://doi.org/10.1016/j.bone.2017.01.024

Falschi P & Marsh D (Eds) (2017) Orthogeriatrics. Springer: Switzerland

Walsh JS (2017), Normal bone physiology, remodelling and its hormonal regulation. Surgery https://doi.org/10.1016/j.mpsur.2017.10.006

1.5.8 How to Self-Assess Learning

- Discuss within the local team if national guidelines for osteoporosis treatment and prevention and fragility fracture prevention are implemented correctly
- Conduct peer-review sessions within the team identifying how team performance impacts on patient outcomes and develop action plans for how practice can be improved
- Undertake assessments contained within online courses listed above.

References

1. Hadjidakis DJ, Androulakis II (2006) Bone Remodeling. Ann N Y Acad Sci 10982(1):385–396
2. Parfitt AM (1982) The coupling of bone formation to bone resorption: critical analysis of the concept and its relevance to the pathogenesis of osteoporosis. Metab Bone Dis Relat Res 4(1):1–6
3. Kloss FR, Gassner R (2006) Bone and aging: effects on the maxillofacial skeleton. Exp Gerontol 41(2):123–129

4. NIH Consensus Development Panel on Osteoporosis Prevention Diagnosis and Therapy (2001) JAMA 285(6):785–795
5. Dempster DW, Raisz LG (2015) Bone physiology: bone cells, modelling and remodelling. In: Holick MF, Nieves JW (eds) Nutrition and bone health. Humana Press, Totowa, pp 37–56
6. Consensus Development Conference (1993) Diagnosis, prophylaxis, and treatment of osteoporosis. Am J Med 94(6):646–650
7. Hernlund E et al (2013) Osteoporosis in the European Union: medical management, epidemiology and economic burden. Arch Osteoporos 8:136
8. Brown JP, Josse RG (2002) Clinical practice guidelines for the diagnosis and management of osteoporosis in Canada. Can Med Assoc J 67(10 Suppl):S1–S34
9. Kanis JA et al (2001) The burden of osteoporotic fractures: a method for setting intervention thresholds. Osteoporos Int 12(5):417–427
10. Rose SH et al (1982) Epidemiologic features of humeral fractures. Clin Orthop Relat Res 168:24–30
11. Nellans KW et al (2012) The epidemiology of distal radius fractures. Hand Clin 28(2):113–125
12. Bukata SV et al (2011) A guide to improving the care of patients with fragility fractures. Geriatr Orthop Surg Rehabil 2(1):5–37
13. Ensrud KE (2013) Epidemiology of fracture risk with advancing age. J Gerontol A Biol Sci Med Sci 8(10):1236–1242
14. International Osteoporosis Foundation. Who's at risk. https://www.iofbonehealth.org/whos-risk
15. Kanis JA et al (2005) Alcohol intake as a risk factor for fracture. Osteoporos Int 16(7):737–742
16. Kanis JA et al (2005) Smoking and fracture risk: a meta-analysis. Osteoporos Int 16(2):155–162
17. Dawson-Hughes B et al (2005) Estimates of optimal vitamin D status. Osteoporos Int 16(7):713–716
18. Wright A (1998) Nursing interventions with advanced osteoporosis. Home Healthc Nurse 16(3):144–151
19. World Health Organization (1994) Assessment of fracture risk and its implication to screening for postmenopausal osteoporosis: Technical report series 843. WHO, Geneva
20. Kanis JA (2002) Diagnosis of osteoporosis and assessment of fracture risk. Lancet 359(9321):1929–1936
21. Kanis JA et al (2008) FRAX™ and the assessment of fracture probability in men and women from the UK. Osteoporos Int 19(4):385–397
22. Fitzpatrick LA (2002) Secondary causes of osteoporosis. Mayo Clin Proc 77(5):453–468
23. Kanis JA et al (2014) The osteoporosis treatment gap. J Bone Miner Res 29(9):1926–1928
24. Netelenbos J et al (2011) Adherence and profile of non-persistence in patients treated for osteoporosis—a large-scale, long-term retrospective study in The Netherlands. Osteoporos Int 22(5):1537–1546

Frailty, Sarcopenia and Falls

2

Andréa Marques and Cármen Queirós

Research confirms that frailty, sarcopenia and falls are strongly correlated [1] and both are predictors of negative health outcomes such as falls, disability, hospitalisation and death [2]. Interventions are necessary to reverse frailty and treat sarcopenia [3] as it has been estimated that, by the year 2025, around 20% of the population in industrial countries will be aged 65 years and over. As the number of older people increases, their needs will become an increasingly important health issue. Reduction in physical function can lead to loss of independence, need for hospital and long-term nursing home care and premature death. The importance of physical, functional, psychological and social factors in realising a healthy old age is recognised by older people, health-care professionals, policy advisors and decision-makers.

This chapter will review the concepts of frailty, sarcopenia and falls as well as the interventions for older people, carried out by nurses and other health-care professionals, that have the potential to positively affect health and functional status and may promote independent functioning of older people with frailty and sarcopenia.

2.1 Learning Outcomes

At the end of the chapter, and following further study, the nurse will be able to:

A. Marques, R.N., M.Sc., Ph.D. (✉)
Rheumatology Department, Centro Hospitalar e Universitário de Coimbra, Coimbra, Portugal
e-mail: amarques@reumahuc.org

C. Queirós
Nursing School of Coimbra, Esenf, Portugal

Escola Superior de Enfermagem do Porto, Porto, Portugal
e-mail: carmenqueiros@gmail.com

K. Hertz, J. Santy-Tomlinson (eds.), *Fragility Fracture Nursing*, Perspectives in Nursing Management and Care for Older Adults, https://doi.org/10.1007/978-3-319-76681-2_2

- Identify individuals with frailty, low muscle mass and depleted strength
- Promote health and prevent ill health in older people with frailty and sarcopenia
- Plan interventions for patients with frailty and sarcopenia
- Educate older people about frailty, sarcopenia and fall prevention
- Promote correct nutrition and physical exercise in frail and sarcopenic patients.

2.2 Frailty

Frailty is a complex societal challenge of an ageing population and has significant repercussions for patient outcomes and health-care utilisation [4]. There is no universally accepted definition [4, 5], but experts agree that it is a clinical syndrome characterised by increased vulnerability and diminished resistance to stressors that can cause functional impairment and increase risks [6, 7]; a minor stress or event such as an accidental fall or infection can worsen a person's health condition and increase dependency and/or mortality. Box 2.1 captures the main concepts in definitions of frailty.

Frailty can be physical or psychological or a combination of the two, with two common models used to explain it: (1) frailty is seen as a syndrome where sarcopenia (loss of muscle with ageing) is the main underlying concept [8] and individuals have at least three of a list of features including; unintentional weight loss, exhaustion, weakness, slowness and reduced physical activity and (2) frailty as the sum of an individual's deficits and non-specific disorders [9] that prevent individuals from launching an effective response to health stressors, leading to adverse health outcomes [6, 10].

Regardless of the perspective, frail patients are at increased risk of adverse health outcomes such as falls, hospitalisation, deterioration of mobility, disability, institutionalisation and death [5, 6, 8], and assessing patients for frailty is an important aspect of the assessment process with several tools available for this. Epidemiological studies [11] have estimated the prevalence of frailty at between 4% and 59%, depending on the population being studied [12], gender (higher in women than men) and age (the oldest have a higher prevalence) [13, 14].

Box 2.1: Frailty Definition

- Clinical syndrome
- Increased vulnerability
- Diminished resistance to stressors
- Can cause functional impairment
- Risk of adverse health outcomes

2.2.1 Assessment

Early diagnosis of frailty can improve care and has an important role in preventing fractures in older adults [15]. All individuals over 70 years of age and all persons with unintentional and significant weight loss should be assessed for frailty [6]. Box 2.2. provides an overview of the most commonly used tools.

A comprehensive review identified 67 instruments for the assessment of frailty. Of these, nine were highly cited: the Physical Frailty Phenotype (PFP—also known as the Fried or CHS Frailty Phenotype), the Deficit Accumulation Index (DAI; also known as Frailty Index), the Gill Frailty Measure, the Frailty/Vigour Assessment, the Clinical Frailty Scale, the Brief Frailty Instrument, the Vulnerable Elders Survey (VES-13), the FRAIL Scale and the Winograd Screening Instrument. The selection of a specific instrument to assess frailty should be based on its purpose, theoretical approach, the validity of the constructs used and its feasibility in the clinical context [16]. More recently, an umbrella review was performed to identify the most valid, reliable and diagnostically accurate frailty screening tools [11], concluding that only a few frailty measures demonstrate these characteristics. Among them, the Frailty Index appeared as the most useful in standard care and community settings. However, the review could not identify an appropriate tool for assessing frailty in EDs, concluding that there is no universally appropriate screening tool for identifying frailty that could be recommended. It is important, however, to provide an overview of the most commonly used tools.

The Physical Frailty Phenotype (PFP, Fried or CHS Frailty Phenotype) was developed following observations of 5000 men and women aged ≥65 years from the Cardiovascular Health Study [8]. This tool defines frailty as the presence of five criteria: weight loss (≥5% of body weight in the previous year), weakness (decreased grip strength), exhaustion (self-reported responses to questions about effort required for activity), slowness on walking (gait speed ≥6–7 s to walk 15 feet) and decreased physical activity (Kcal spent per week: males expending <383 Kcal and females <270 Kcal) [8]. The assessment requires specialised equipment for grip strength measurement and involves patient participation to calculate gait speed. The PFP also facilitates identifying "pre-frailty"; one or two of the criteria for frailty are present.

The Deficit Accumulation or Frailty Index [9] is based on the individual's accumulated burden of illnesses, functional and cognitive decline and other health related deficits that, together, provide a flexible measurement of frailty. Deficits are measured by answering medical and functional related questions, allowing a frailty index to be quantified; the higher the number of deficits, the higher the frailty score. An assessment that identifies a score of 30–40 deficits has been shown to be able to predict adverse health outcomes [9, 17]. One advantage of using this tool, versus PFP, is that it does not require a patient interview or exam, as the information can be retrieved from health records.

Some other instruments commonly used to assess frailty are quicker to use and, therefore, easier for nurses to apply; e.g. the Clinical Frailty Scale, FRAIL Scale and Study of Osteoporotic Fractures (SOF) frailty tool. The Clinical Frailty Scale uses pictographs and descriptors to categorise between very fit (−1) and severely frail (−7). The assessment involves self-reporting (with no need for face-to-face examination) of comorbidities and the need for assistance with activities of daily living [18, 19]. The scale is composed of five questions with "FRAIL" as an acronym: F = fatigue, R = resistance, A = ambulation, I = illnesses and L = loss of weight [20, 21]; three or more positive answerers indicate frailty, and one or two positive answerers indicate pre-frailty. The Study of Osteoporotic Fractures (SOF) frailty tool assesses frailty according to three characteristics: loss of 5% of body weight in the last year, inability to stand up from a chair five times without the use of arms and feeling full of energy; two positive answers to the first and second items and/or a negative to the last one classifies the person as frail [22].

Box 2.2: Frailty Assessment

- Individuals older than 70 years
- Individuals with unintentional and substantial weight loss (≥5%)
- The most common assessment tools are:
  - Physical Frailty Phenotype
  - Frailty Index
- Other instruments commonly used which are quicker and easier to adopt are:
  - Clinical Frailty Scale
  - FRAIL Scale
  - Study of Osteoporotic Fractures (SOF) frailty tool

2.2.2 Interventions

Health-care interventions can help to improve the degree of frailty over time [6]. Evidence relates to four possible interventions (Box 2.3): (1) exercise (aerobic and resistance), (2) calorie and protein supplementation, (3) vitamin D supplementation and (4) reduction of polypharmacy [6, 14, 21]:

- Planned exercise can develop muscle strength and improve physical performance and functionality [23] as well as decrease depression and fear of falling [6]. A mix of specifically prescribed aerobic and resistance exercises improves frailty and is effective in preventing its adverse outcomes [24, 25]. One systematic review found that an exercise programme, continued three times a week for 30–45 min per session for approximately 5 months, had positive impact [26].
- In frail older people with significant weight loss, it is essential to identify the cause (Chap. 8). Dietary calorific supplementation has been shown to be successful in achieving weight gain and reducing complications in malnourished individuals [27]. Protein supplementation of 15 g of protein twice a day over 24 weeks improves muscle strength and physical performance [28], while oral nutritional supplements provide additional protein and calories.

- Vitamin D supplementation can play a role in preventing or treating frailty by enhancing balance and maintaining muscle strength [29] but, while this is likely to be beneficial for frail older people, there have been no large-scale studies that have confirmed this to be the case on its own [6].
- Undertaking a medication review and considering side effects, interactions and consequences for frailty is essential. Medication review and reduction of polypharmacy have also been advocated as an option for improving outcomes, especially in reducing mortality, hospital admissions and falls [30].

These four interventions should be considered following frailty assessment so that they can be individually tailored to target specific identified problems and needs [31].

Box 2.3: Interventions
- Exercise (aerobic and resistance)
- Caloric and protein supplementation
- Vitamin D supplementation
- Reduction of polypharmacy

2.3 Sarcopenia

Changes in body composition occur with normal physiological ageing [32]; usually, body weight increases during adulthood and peaks at the age of 65 years in women and 54 years in men [33]. Muscle mass is lost at a rate of approximately 8% per decade between the ages 50 and 70 years; then weight loss is coupled with an accelerated loss of muscle mass, reaching a rate of 15% each decade [33]. The overall prevalence of sarcopenia is reported to be 10% [34]; with the continued increase in the older population, sarcopenia is becoming a serious global public health problem.

Sarcopenia is associated with the ageing process [35]; loss of muscle mass and strength, which in turn affects balance, gait and overall ability to perform tasks of daily living, are hallmarks of this disease that is also a powerful predictor of disability [36]. The risk of disability is 1.5–4.6 times higher in older people with sarcopenia than in those with normal muscle. These common age-related changes in skeletal muscle are major causes of impaired physical function in older adults, contributing to impaired mobility, falls and hospitalisation. The causes of sarcopenia are multifactorial and can include muscle disuse, changing endocrine function, chronic diseases, inflammation, insulin resistance and nutritional deficiencies [38]; reductions in testosterone and oestrogen that accompany ageing appear to accelerate its development [39].

2.3.1 Screening and Assessment for Sarcopenia

Sarcopenia, like many other health conditions, is asymptomatic in its initial stages, when interventions can best prevent the adverse health outcomes [40]. Screening is currently not a routine aspect of clinical practice, partly because of the lack of appropriate screening strategies [41]. An ideal screening test should be cheap, acceptable and easily implementable without requiring additional training [42]. Several expert groups have convened with the goal of establishing a consensus about diagnostic criteria for sarcopenia [43–46]; a common theme is that diagnosis of sarcopenia should include identification of both low muscle mass and poor muscle function, indicated by either low muscle strength or impaired physical performance, such as slow gait speed. The European Working Group on Sarcopenia in Older People (EWGSOP) consensus outlined an algorithm to aid the screening and diagnosis of sarcopenia. Box 2.4 shows the diagnostic criteria. Patients with gait speeds of 0.8 m/s or less should then undergo a second performance assessment, such as grip strength. Those meeting the criteria for low grip strength should be assessed by DXA (Chap. 1) or bioelectrical impedance analysis (BIA) to confirm the presence or absence of sarcopenia [44].

Box 2.4: Diagnostic Criteria for Sarcopenia

Sarcopenia should be considered in patients with presence of criteria 1 plus criteria 2 or 3:

Criteria 1: Low muscle mass

DXA >2 SD below mean of the younger adults:

- Men <7.26 kg/m^2
- Women <5.5 kg/m^2

Lowest 20% of the distribution of appendicular skeletal mass (ASM) in a normative population (aged 65 years and older)

- Men <7.23 kg/m^2
- Women <5.67 kg/m^2

Lowest 20% distribution of the residual of ASM adjusting for height and fat mass

- Men <2.29
- Women: <1.73

BIA >2 SD below mean (SMI) of the younger adults

- Men <8.87 kg/m^2
- Women <6.42 kg/m^2

Criteria 2: Low grip strength

- Men: <30 kg
- Women: <20 kg

Criteria 3: Low physical performance

- Short Performance Battery (SPPB) ≤8
- Gait speed <0.8 m/s

2.3.2 The Clinical Consequences of Sarcopenia

Osteoporosis predicts the future risk of fracture; and sarcopenia is a powerful predictor of future disability [32]. Reduced muscle mass and strength are also associated with lower bone mineral density [47, 48], consistent with the "mechanostat" theory of bone loss due to reduced forces of muscle on bone [49]. In fact, sarcopenia may contribute to falls and, as a consequence, increase fracture risk [50, 51]. Hence, not surprisingly, there is evidence that low muscle mass and strength are associated with fractures [51]. Several studies have confirmed associations between low muscle mass, future functional decline and physical disability [2]. Physical inactivity or decreased physical activity is part of the underlying mechanisms of sarcopenia, so physical activity is important in reversing or modifying it. Several interventions have been proposed for the treatment of this loss of muscle and strength, but exercise is central. Sarcopenia has also been linked to higher hospitalisation rates, increased morbidity and mortality [52, 53]. Sarcopenia may also be associated with metabolic and cardiovascular diseases such as diabetes, dyslipidaemia and hypertension [32].

2.3.3 Interventions to Prevent Sarcopenia

It is better to prevent progressive loss of skeletal muscle mass, strength and function rather than try to restore it later, so preventive strategies should be initiated early, before loss of skeletal muscle mass and strength occurs.

Exercise interventions have the most significant improvement in sarcopenia. The benefits of physical activity in the elderly population include lower mortality and functional independence (Chap. 6). There are four specific categories of recommended exercise: (1) aerobic exercise, (2) progressive resistance exercise, (3) flexibility exercise and (4) balance training [3].

Nutrition is also important in preventing and reversing sarcopenia (Chap. 7). Increasing age is associated with reduced appetite and early satiety, resulting in many older people failing to meet the recommended daily dietary allowance (RDA) for protein, which has important implications for skeletal muscles [54]. Older adults will require higher dietary protein (up to 1.2 g/kg/day) to counteract age-related changes in protein metabolism and higher catabolic state associated with chronic or acute diseases [55].

It is the combination of exercise and nutrition interventions that is the key to preventing, treating and slowing down the progression of sarcopenia [54]. Pharmaceutical agents are under investigation but with no current proven benefit. Pharmacological agents such as myostatin inhibitors, testosterone, angiotensin-converting enzyme inhibitors and ghrelin-modulating agents are being investigated to treat sarcopenia, but there is inadequate evidence to support their use. Low serum vitamin D levels are associated with reduced muscle strength, and it has also been demonstrated that a dose-response relationship exists between serum levels and muscle health. If serum levels are low, vitamin D should be replaced with replenishment dosages ranging from 700 to 1000 IU/day [56].

Box 2.5: Multiple Factors That Contribute Collectively to Frailty, Sarcopenia and Falls

Potentially treatable:

- Social factors including social isolation, living alone
- Lack of access to transport
- Elder abuse
- Poverty and food insecurity
- Failure to provide for ethnic food preference
- Inability to prepare and cook meals or to feed self
- Inability to shop
- Alcoholism

Medical:

- Thyroid disease
- Cardiac failure
- Gastrointestinal disease affecting absorption: anorexia (antibiotics/digoxin), early satiety (anticholinergic drugs), reduced feeding ability (such as sedatives/psychotropics), dysphagia (NSAIDs), constipation (opiates/diuretics), diarrhoea (laxatives/antibiotics), hypermetabolism (thyroxin)
- Sensory impairment—vision/hearing
- Oral problem, e.g. poorly fitting dentures
- Swallowing problem/dysphagia, thickened diet
- Poorly managed pain or constipation

More difficult to treat:

- Medical factors
- Loss of taste and smell, restricted diets
- Cognition—dementia
- Catabolism
- Gastritis
- Cancer
- Mood—depression, paranoia
- Medications/polypharmacy

Implementing interventions for frailty and sarcopenia has several challenges and barriers. A systematic review demonstrated that older people believe that exercise is unnecessary or, even, potentially harmful [58]. Others recognise the benefits of exercise but report a range of barriers to participation in exercise interventions. Raising awareness is important to enhance exercise participation among older people and to prevent sarcopenia.

Another barrier that needs to be considered in planning long-term strategies to prevent and treat sarcopenia in older people is the financial ability to attend exercise programmes [59]. Factors such as access to food, finances and social isolation may all impact on an older person's ability to obtain optimal food intake.

2.4 The Link Between Frailty, Sarcopenia and Falls

Falls in older people are associated with multicomponent impairments, particularly of muscle function, balance and cognition, so are best understood as resulting from complex system failure as part of the frailty syndrome in the presence of sarcopenia [57]. Falls and fall prevention are considered in more detail in Chap. 3. Box 2.5 provides an overview of the multiple factors that contribute collectively to frailty, sarcopenia and falls, which include cellular and tissue changes, as well as environmental and behavioural factors.

2.5 Suggested Further Study

Search for information and online programmes on the impact of ageing on older people:

- http://aginginmotion.org/
- https://nos.org.uk/for-health-professionals/
- https://www.cme.nof.org/

Talk with patients, carers and other staff about the things they feel that lead to and prevent frailty, sarcopenia and falls. Reflect on what these conversations suggest about how practice might be developed to improve mobility outcomes by involving patients.

2.6 How to Self-Assess Learning

- Seek advice and mentorship from other expert clinicians.
- Meet with specialists and other members of the team to keep up to date on new evidence and disseminate it to colleagues.
- Search on a regular basis about recent new practices, guidance, knowledge or evidence.

References

1. Reijnierse EM et al (2016) Common ground? the concordance of sarcopenia and frailty definitions. J Am Med Dir Assoc 17(4):371.e7–371.12
2. Beaudart C et al (2017) Health outcomes of sarcopenia: a systematic review and meta-analysis. PLoS One 12(1):e0169548

3. Lozano-Montoya I et al (2017) Nonpharmacological interventions to treat physical frailty and sarcopenia in older patients: a systematic overview—the SENATOR Project ONTOP Series. Clin Interv Aging 12:721–740
4. Sutton JL et al (2016) Psychometric properties of multicomponent tools designed to assess frailty in older adults: a systematic review. BMC Geriatr 16:55
5. Lohman MC et al (2017) Depression and frailty: concurrent risks for adverse health outcomes. Aging Ment Health 21(4):399–408
6. Morley JE et al (2013) Frailty consensus: a call to action. J Am Med Dir Assoc 14(6):392–397
7. Rodriguez-Manas L et al (2013) Searching for an operational definition of frailty: a Delphi method based consensus statement: the frailty operative definition-consensus conference project. J Gerontol A Biol Sci Med Sci 68(1):62–67
8. Fried LP et al (2001) Frailty in older adults: evidence for a phenotype. J Gerontol A Biol Sci Med Sci 56(3):M146–MM57
9. Rockwood K, Mitnitski A (2007) Frailty in relation to the accumulation of deficits. J Gerontol A Biol Sci Med Sci 62(7):722–727
10. Chowdhury R et al (2017) Frailty and chronic kidney disease: a systematic review. Arch Gerontol Geriatr 68:135–142
11. Apóstolo J et al (2017) Predicting risk and outcomes for frail older adults: an umbrella review of frailty screening tools. JBI Database System Rev Implement Rep 15(4):1154–1208
12. Wilson MG et al (2015) Interventions for preventing, delaying the onset, or decreasing the burden of frailty: an overview of systematic reviews. Syst Rev 4:128
13. Collard RM et al (2012) Prevalence of frailty in community-dwelling older persons: a systematic review. J Am Geriatr Soc 60(8):1487–1492
14. Tello-Rodriguez T, Varela-Pinedo L (2016) Frailty in older adults: detection, community-based intervention, and decision-making in the management of chronic illnesses. Rev Peru Med Exp Salud Publica 33(2):328–334
15. Wei Chen K, Chang S-F (2017) Frailty was related with fracture: a systematic review. Int J Nurs Health Sci 3(1):1–4
16. Buta BJ et al (2016) Frailty assessment instruments: systematic characterization of the uses and contexts of highly-cited instruments. Ageing Res Rev 26:53–61
17. Searle SD et al (2008) A standard procedure for creating a frailty index. BMC Geriatr 8:24
18. Juma S (2016) Clinical Frailty Scale in an Acute Medicine Unit: a Simple Tool That Predicts Length of Stay. Can Geriatr J 19(2):34–39
19. Rockwood K et al (2005) A global clinical measure of fitness and frailty in elderly people. CMAJ 173(5):489–489
20. Morley JE et al (2012) A simple frailty questionnaire (FRAIL) predicts outcomes in middle aged African Americans. J Nutr Health Aging 16(7):601–608
21. Morley JE (2014) Frailty screening comes of age. J Nutr Health Aging 18(5):453–454
22. Silva J et al (2017) Impact of insomnia on self-perceived health in the elderly. Arq Neuropsiquiatr 75(5):277–281
23. Cruz-Jentoft AJ (2014) Prevalence of and interventions for sarcopenia in ageing adults: a systematic review. Report of the International Sarcopenia Initiative (EWGSOP and IWGS). Age Ageing 43(6):748–759
24. Marzetti E et al (2017) Physical activity and exercise as countermeasures to physical frailty and sarcopenia. Aging Clin Exp Res 29(1):35–42
25. Cesari M et al (2015) A physical activity intervention to treat the frailty syndrome in older persons-results from the LIFE-P study. J Gerontol A Biol Sci Med Sci 70(2):216–222
26. Theou O et al (2011) The effectiveness of exercise interventions for the management of frailty: a systematic review. J Aging Res 569194
27. Milne AC et al (2009) Protein and energy supplementation in elderly people at risk from malnutrition. Cochrane Database Syst Rev. 2009;(2):CD003288. doi: https://doi.org/10.1002/14651858.CD003288.pub3.
28. Tieland M et al (2012) Protein supplementation improves physical performance in frail elderly people: a randomized, double-blind, placebo-controlled trial. J Am Med Dir Assoc 13(8):720–726

29. Montero-Odasso M, Duque G (2005) Vitamin D in the aging musculoskeletal system: an authentic strength preserving hormone. Mol Aspects Med 26(3):203–219
30. Romera L et al (2014) Effectiveness of a primary care based multifactorial intervention to improve frailty parameters in the elderly: a randomised clinical trial: rationale and study design. BMC Geriatr 14:125
31. Cameron ID et al (2013) A multifactorial interdisciplinary intervention reduces frailty in older people: randomized trial. BMC Med 11:65
32. Shaw SC (2017) Epidemiology of sarcopenia: determinants throughout the lifecourse. Calcif Tissue Int 101(3):229–247
33. Yu S et al (2014) Sarcopenia in older people. Int J Evid Based Healthc 12(4):227–243
34. Shafiee G et al (2017) Prevalence of sarcopenia in the world: a systematic review and meta-analysis of general population studies. J Diabetes Metab Disord 16:21
35. Steen B (1988) Body Composition and Aging. Nutr Rev 46(2):45–51
36. Morley JE (2016) Frailty and Sarcopenia: the new geriatric giants. Rev Invest Clin 68(2):59–67
37. Janssen I et al (2004) The healthcare costs of sarcopenia in the United States. J Am Geriatr Soc 52(1):80–85
38. Janssen I (2011) The epidemiology of sarcopenia. Clin Geriatr Med 27(3):355–363
39. Joseph C et al (2005) Role of endocrine-immune dysregulation in osteoporosis, sarcopenia, frailty and fracture risk. Mol Aspects Med 26(3):181–201
40. McLean RR, Kiel DP (2015) Developing consensus criteria for sarcopenia: an update. J Bone Miner Res 30(4):588–592
41. Studenski SA et al (2014) The FNIH sarcopenia project: rationale, study description, conference recommendations, and final estimates. J Gerontol A Biol Sci Med Sci 69(5):547–558
42. Fields MM, Chevlen E (2006) Screening for disease: making evidence-based choices. Clin J Oncol Nurs 10(1):73–76
43. Muscaritoli M et al (2010) Consensus definition of sarcopenia, cachexia and pre-cachexia: joint document elaborated by Special Interest Groups (SIG). Cachexia-anorexia in chronic wasting diseases" and "nutrition in geriatrics". Clin Nutr 29(2):154–159
44. Cruz-Jentoft AJ et al (2010) Sarcopenia: European consensus on definition and diagnosis: report of the European Working Group on Sarcopenia in Older People. Age Ageing 39(4):412–423
45. Fielding RA et al (2011) Sarcopenia: an undiagnosed condition in older adults. Current consensus definition: prevalence, etiology, and consequences. International working group on sarcopenia. J Am Med Dir Assoc 12(4):249–256
46. Morley JE et al (2011) Sarcopenia with limited mobility: an international consensus. J Am Med Dir Assoc 12(6):403–409
47. Proctor DN et al (2000) Relative influence of physical activity, muscle mass and strength on bone density. Osteoporos Int 11(11):944–952
48. Singh H et al (2017) Relationship between muscle performance and DXA-derived bone parameters in community-dwelling older adults. J Musculoskelet Neuronal Interact 17(2):50–58
49. Frost HM (2003) Bone's mechanostat: a 2003 update. Anat Rec A Discov Mol Cell Evol Biol 275(2):1081–1101
50. Landi F et al (2012) Sarcopenia as a risk factor for falls in elderly individuals: results from the ilSIRENTE study. Clin Nutr 31(5):652–658
51. Cederholm T et al (2013) Sarcopenia and fragility fractures. Eur J Phys Rehabil Med 49(1):111–117
52. Oakland K et al (2016) Systematic review and meta-analysis of the association between frailty and outcome in surgical patients. Ann R Coll Surg Engl 98(2):80–85
53. Wang SY et al (2013) Not just specific diseases: systematic review of the association of geriatric syndromes with hospitalization or nursing home admission. Arch Gerontol Geriatr 57(1):16–26
54. Deutz NE et al (2014) Protein intake and exercise for optimal muscle function with aging: recommendations from the ESPEN Expert Group. Clin Nutr 33(6):929–936
55. Bauer J et al (2013) Evidence-based recommendations for optimal dietary protein intake in older people: a position paper from the PROT-AGE Study Group. J Am Med Dir Assoc 14(8):542–559

56. Bischoff Ferrari HA (2009) Validated treatments and therapeutic perspectives regarding nutritherapy. J Nutr Health Aging 13(8):737–741
57. Boirie Y (2009) Physiopathological mechanism of sarcopenia. J Nutr Health Aging 13(8):717–723
58. Franco MR et al (2015) Older people's perspectives on participation in physical activity: a systematic review and thematic synthesis of qualitative literature. Br J Sports Med 49(19):1268–1276
59. Freiberger E (2011) Physical activity, exercise, and sarcopenia—future challenges. Wien Med Wochenschr 161(17-18):416–425

3 Falls and Secondary Fracture Prevention

Julie Santy-Tomlinson, Robyn Speerin, Karen Hertz, Ana Cruz Tochon-Laruaz, and Marsha van Oostwaard

The most common cause of fractures in the elderly is falling, usually from standing height, and falling is the leading cause of hospitalisation due to accidental injury, with significant risk of death in the following year due to complications [1]. Low bone density due to osteoporosis or osteopenia means that falls easily result in fractures, even when the fall dynamics are relatively mild, as discussed in Chap. 1. These are often referred to as 'fragility', 'osteoporotic' or 'minimal trauma' fractures and most commonly occur in those over the age of 50 years [2], the same population at risk of osteoporosis.

The cumulative risk of fragility fractures is reported to be 51% for women and 20% for men [3], representing a significant challenge to health services. Up to 5% of falls result in fracture and 1% in hip fracture, but it is estimated that the incidence of hip fracture could increase by as much as 66% by 2021 [4]. A hip

J. Santy-Tomlinson (✉)
Division of Nursing, Midwifery and Social Work, School of Health Sciences, Faculty of Biology, Medicine and Health, The University of Manchester, Manchester, UK
e-mail: Julie.santy-tomlinson@manchester.ac.uk

R. Speerin
Musculoskeletal Network, NSW Agency for Clinical Innovation, Chatswood, NSW, Australia
e-mail: Robyn.speerin@health.nsw.gov.au

K. Hertz
Specialised Division, University Hospital of North Midlands, Stoke-on-Trent, Staffordshire, UK
e-mail: Karen.hertz@uhnm.nhs.uk

A. C. Tochon-Laruaz
Division of Bone Diseases, Geneva University Hospitals, Geneva, Switzerland
e-mail: ANA.CRUZ@HCUGE.CH

M. van Oostwaard
Màxima Medisch Centrum, Eindhoven, The Netherlands
e-mail: M.vanOostwaard@mmc.nl

K. Hertz, J. Santy-Tomlinson (eds.), *Fragility Fracture Nursing*, Perspectives in Nursing Management and Care for Older Adults, https://doi.org/10.1007/978-3-319-76681-2_3

fracture has the greatest impact on the individual of all fragility fractures and is associated with the worst morbidity, mortality and functional ability outcomes from fractures [5]. It leads to extensive hospitalisation and can result in major complications and death [6]. Even minor fractures, such as those of the wrist, can lead to significant impairment and early mortality, independent of any contributing co-morbidities [7]. Older people who are healthier and more active can sustain fractures much later in life, making their care more complex [8]. Hence, there is an imperative to support successful primary and secondary prevention of falls and osteoporosis.

The prevention of falls is central to preventing fractures; their impact is far-reaching and includes physical, psychological and social effects. Falls and fear of falling can lead to impaired mobility and fear of further falls resulting in isolation, reduced self-esteem, anxiety and depression; so it is the impact of a fall or multiple falls that must be considered, even without a fracture. Those whose low-impact fall results in a fracture need holistic, person-centred assessment and secondary fracture prevention, identifying osteoporosis and initiating and sustaining treatment as well as preventing future falls. Models of care for secondary or refracture prevention have been implemented internationally over the past 15–20 years and are commonly known as 'Fracture Liaison Services'. These services aim to identify people who have sustained a fragility fracture and help them to gain access to their required treatment and support to sustain therapies known to reduce the incidence of further fractures. Treatment and supportive follow-up are known to prevent at least 50% of projected subsequent fractures but, despite the hallmark of having had a fragility fracture, many with osteoporosis remain undiagnosed and untreated [9]. This chapter aims to discuss the prevention of falls and secondary fractures through evidence-based interventions and services.

3.1 Learning Outcomes

At the end of this chapter and following further study, the nurse will be able to:

- Identify the causes of and risk factors for falling
- Employ evidence-based nursing interventions for the prevention of falls
- Instigate and coordinate falls prevention strategies in people who sustain fragility fractures
- Define the concept of secondary fracture prevention
- Explain the need for coordinated secondary fracture prevention through pathways and models of care such as Fracture Liaison Services
- Discuss the role of the practitioner in secondary fracture prevention and Fracture Liaison Services
- Outline how secondary refracture prevention services can be developed, implemented and evaluated.

3.2 Falls

Falls predominantly occur in people over the age of 65 years. Eighty percent of fractures of the axial skeleton result from a fall [6]. Approximately 30% of older people fall at least once per year, depending on age, gender, country and ethnicity, increasing to 50% of those over the age of 80 years, especially those living in residential carc facilities. Half of those who fall do so repeatedly. Falls are multifactorial and research has reported numerous causes and risk factors in older people [10].

3.2.1 Causes of and Risk Factors for Falls

Understanding the reasons why older people fall is an important part of assessment leading to evidence-based intervention and should be an integral part of the comprehensive assessment process discussed in Chap. 4. Many research teams have investigated the factors most likely to lead to an individual falling:

Intrinsic factors: person-specific, including characteristics of the individual and their medical conditions such as sarcopenia and other age-related conditions. These include age, gender, gait, fitness, balance, strength and aerobic fitness, vertigo and dizziness, impaired vision and hearing, cognitive impairment, cardiovascular disease, medications (particularly psychotropic) and depression [11].

Extrinsic factors: environmental factors that present fall hazards in the home and external environment such as footwear and clothing, home lighting, flooring, tripping hazards, lack of grab bars and unstable furniture [11].

3.2.2 Screening and Assessment

The purpose of screening and assessment is to facilitate interventions that will help reduce the incidence of falls and their consequences. The terms screening and assessment tend to be used interchangeably, but screening determines if assessment is required, and assessment involves gathering more detailed information needed to direct a prevention plan that meets individual needs and wishes. Many tools are available to help practitioners undertake screening and assessment for falls.

All older people, whether living in the community or in residential care, should be regularly screened for risk of falling, so that detailed assessment and multidisciplinary interventions can be offered. The most important screening approach is to routinely ask all older people presenting for health care if they have fallen in the past year [12] followed by asking about the frequency and nature of their fall/s. Observing the way that older people move is a simple way to identify those who are at risk; look for slow, asymmetrical, shuffling and unstable gait. If the person struggles to stand from a chair, it indicates a falls risk because of reduced muscle strength. These observations can identify those who require interventions for sarcopenia (described in Chap. 2). Examples of validated screening tools are listed in Box 3.1

Box 3.1: Examples of Screening Tools for Falls in Older People

Modified falls efficacy scale [13]: a 14-item patient-reported measure regarding their confidence in activities of daily living.

Timed Up and Go test (TUG) [14]: the person is timed getting up from a chair, walking 2 metres, walking back to the chair and sitting down. The time taken indicates the falls risk [10].

Thirty-second chair stand [15]: focused on functional ability related to repeated standing from a chair.

Tinetti balance assessment tool [16]: detailed assessment of balance and gait focused on chronic disabilities.

3.2.3 Falls Prevention Strategies

Falls prevention strategies are complex. The most appropriate prevention interventions to reduce fractures depend on the risk profile [6] and, for those in hospital, the place of planned discharge is an important consideration. Interventions may be multifactorial with multiple components aiming to address individual risk factors [14]. Strategies may include:

- Environmental adaptations
- Exercise programmes—strength, balance and cardiovascular training
- Assessment of vision and referral
- Medication review and modification
- Review of feet and footwear.

3.2.3.1 Environment

Most falls occur in the home [18]. Whether the person lives at home, or is hospitalised and is likely to be discharged home, an assessment of the home is essential in identifying environmental changes needed as part of a multicomponent strategy. Assessment should be undertaken by a health/social care professional with the skills to identify problems and recommend adaptations. A home assessment will capture issues relating to flooring, lighting, unstable furniture, access to toilet and bathroom, tripping hazards, safety of cooking facilities and other aspects of the home and garden which may contribute to falls. A plan for adaptation of the home can involve, for example, simple measures such as removing rugs and other tripping hazards, rearranging furniture and providing simple aids such as commodes and raised toilet seats. More complex adaptations can include the installation of grab rails, alarm systems and other building adaptations [6]. Residential care facilities need to be environmentally designed with these principles in mind.

3.2.3.2 Exercise

Exercise strategies for falls prevention focus on balance, strength training and aerobic fitness to improve the individuals' postural stability and ability to resist falling. Group and home-based exercise programmes can reduce the rate of and risk of falls [19] along with some effect on fear of falling [20]. Supervised exercise sessions are recommended at the outset to work towards improved strength and stability before embarking on a self-led home exercise programme [6]. Physiotherapists or exercise physiologists are ideal team members to supervise regular training sessions that include different exercise modalities [21].

3.2.3.3 Vision

Visual impairment is a common contributor to falls risk; affecting balance, ability to avoid obstacles, judgement of distance and spatial awareness [11]. Formal assessment of vision should be offered, along with reduction of environmental hazards and support for the individual's own coping mechanisms.

3.2.3.4 Medication Review

The use of multiple medications in older people can be a significant cause of falls, particularly psychotropic drugs [22]. As part of the CGA process discussed in Chap. 4, a review of medication use is essential. NICE [12] recommends that, with specialist advice, those taking psychotropic medications, in particular, should have their dose reviewed or discontinued. A review of cardiac medications should also be undertaken so medications can be reduced, if required, with as little cardiovascular risk as is possible. Hypotension is a common cause of falling, but some medications are known to improve quality of life in those with heart failure. While hypotension is common in heart failure, with no resultant dizziness, these medications should be titrated only with judicious cardiology expertise in order to provide the person with as much quality of life while living with heart failure but to also reduce falls risk.

3.2.3.5 Footwear and Foot Care

Modification of footwear and care of feet is a fundamental aspect of falls prevention. Foot pain and weakness, reduced range of motion, deformity and inappropriate footwear are all risk factors [23]. Many people at risk of falls will have type 2 diabetes, so it is important to help them understand the need for inspection of feet daily, including the soles of the feet, especially when starting an exercise programme, in order to identify potential ulcers or broken skin at the earliest possible stage of development. All older people should be advised to wear supportive shoes rather than wear slippers or walk in socks in the home [24]. The podiatrist is an important member of the MDT and needs to be consulted for expert management when foot problems are identified [23].

3.2.3.6 Fear of Falling

Fear of falling is a psychological consequence of previous falls. Fear leads to anxiety, loss of confidence and isolation due to decreased activity, and this increases frailty and the likelihood of further falls [25]. Practitioners recognise fear of falling that as reluctance to mobilise. It is revealed as anxiousness when asked to try mobilisation, along with clutching and grabbing. This is a complex problem that needs a multifactorial, multidisciplinary approach. Although there is limited evidence relating to specific interventions to reduce fear of falling [26], practitioners can mitigate the effects of fear by the use of strategies that include gradually and sensitively reintroducing the person to remobilisation using realistic short- and long-term goal setting, supporting attempts to mobilise with encouragement and use of mobility aids, allowing plenty of time for completion of activities and offering plenty of opportunities to practise a little and often.

3.2.3.7 Falls Pathways and Guidelines

Falls prevention pathways and guidelines have been developed to guide effective assessment and the planning, implementation and evaluation of multicomponent interventions. Local guidelines will help to guide practice. These pathways and guidelines facilitate collaboration and integration to bring emergency services, acute, secondary and primary care services together to coordinate care. The inclusion of people who require the pathway (and their families or carers) in decision-making is facilitated through education and information about what can be achieved through the activities of falls prevention [12].

3.3 Secondary Fracture Prevention

Sustaining a fragility fracture is the signal that more fractures will occur, so health care that is known to prevent greater than 40% of the refractures must be instigated [27]. Unfortunately health-care systems across the globe often fail to provide this care because:

1. No one professional group takes responsibility for identifying and treating this patient group.
2. As people with fragility fracture are not advised of their high potential of having osteoporosis, they never report this condition in surveys, so the subsequent population numbers of those with osteoporosis are reported erroneously to be low.
3. Coding in health records is poor due to clinical teams not using terms in their medical records that inform the coder to report fragility fractures.
4. A lack of international codes to use, even when the fragility fracture is identified.

This results in health systems being unaware of the need for action and failing to implement secondary prevention services that reduce refracture rates, improve the quality of life of those who sustain fragility fractures and reduce the mortality that is directly attributable to any fragility fracture, not just hip fractures [7].

It has been estimated that about 20% of people sustaining a fragility fracture gain access to secondary prevention care despite the evidence internationally that reveals that 'Fracture Liaison Services', a systematic approach to secondary prevention, result in fewer refractures and significant cost savings [28].

3.3.1 Fracture Prevention Services and Guidelines

The International Osteoporosis Foundation (IOF) has developed 'Capture the Fracture', a best practice framework that defines essential elements of service delivery and evaluation of Fracture Liaison Services (FLS) [28]. The aim of these services is to have processes in place that ensure each person who sustains a fragility fracture of any part of the skeleton:

- Is identified as requiring organised care that aims to prevent the next fracture
- Understands the need to improve their bone health and how this is achieved through their efforts in tandem with their health-care team
- Has access to investigation of their bone health and understands precipitating factors that may make them susceptible to osteoporosis and further fractures
- Has local access to required medical and other care such as falls prevention services and exercise programmes
- Their health teams in primary and secondary care collaborate to ensure person-/family-centred care working in tandem
- Is followed-up regularly long-term to support adherence to treatment with periodical medical review to ensure their treatment remains appropriate for them.

The FLS must be delivered in a multidisciplinary environment with all team members using behaviour change methodologies to support patient-centred care with self-management support as the key intervention.

Services can be based in primary or secondary care settings but must include a coordinator-based system led by what is internationally referred to as the Fracture Liaison Coordinator [39]. The Fracture Liaison Coordinator, commonly a senior nurse or physiotherapist, provides support and understanding of the needs of those sustaining fragility fractures, helping them understand the need for assessment and ongoing treatment. The coordinator works closely with a medical practitioner who undertakes medical assessment and prescribes treatment. The medical practitioner can also be from a range of medical specialities including, but not limited to; orthopaedic surgery and medicine, primary care and specialist physicians, rheumatology, endocrinology, geriatrics, rehabilitation and pain medicine. In some areas, nurse practitioners work within a designated scope of practice in tandem with medical officers to undertake some of the medical assessment and prescribing of treatment regimens.

The team approach to care of people receiving care within an FLS ensures best practice care is provided and facilitates collaboration between primary care providers such as physicians, falls prevention and radiology services and secondary care providers such as orthopaedic and emergency care teams. This approach ensures a supportive environment for the person who has had a fragility fracture and allows seamless care and continuity of education about bone health and co-morbidities.

Responsibilities of the Fracture Liaison Coordinator include:

- Being the link between people who access the service and the multidisciplinary team and health service in the hospital, but particularly in the community and especially primary care physicians, as well as facilitating and agreeing formal communication processes
- Coordinating a steering group to guide the service development over time
- Creating and maintaining records of assessment, treatment and outcomes with cooperation of the multidisciplinary team members
- Leading the development, implementation and evaluation of quality improvement projects to ensure ongoing improvements of the service as required
- Supporting and encouraging team members to extend their knowledge in contemporary fracture prevention through self-study and education.

Outcomes from different models of care vary; the more intensive the model of care, the better the health outcomes; Ganda et al. [9] conducted a review of the various reported models of care and found that the more intensive the model of care, the more cost-effective it was with improved quality of life through refracture prevention (see Table 3.1). This has also been shown by Nakayama et al. [27], who examined a FLS at a hospital where an intensive model of care is used. Comparing that hospital's fragility fracture presentations to those of a hospital where no FLS was in place revealed that there were 40% less hip fracture presentations than at the no service site.

Table 3.1 Common models of Fracture Liaison Service (FLS)

FLS model type	Interventions provided within the model of care	Outcomes
A	Intensive service with all interventions, the responsibility of the team	Most effective across all care needs for people who sustain a fragility fracture and is cost-effective with the most refractures prevented
B	All interventions except treatment initiation—the responsibility of the patient's general practitioner	Not as effective as type A but more effective than health education alone
C	Health education only provided with handover to the general practitioner from a physician either through written or phone call communication	Little or no effect on initiation of effective treatment known to reduce the incidence of refracture
D	Health education provided. There is no physician contact with the person's general practitioner	No effect on initiation of effective treatment known to reduce the incidence of refracture

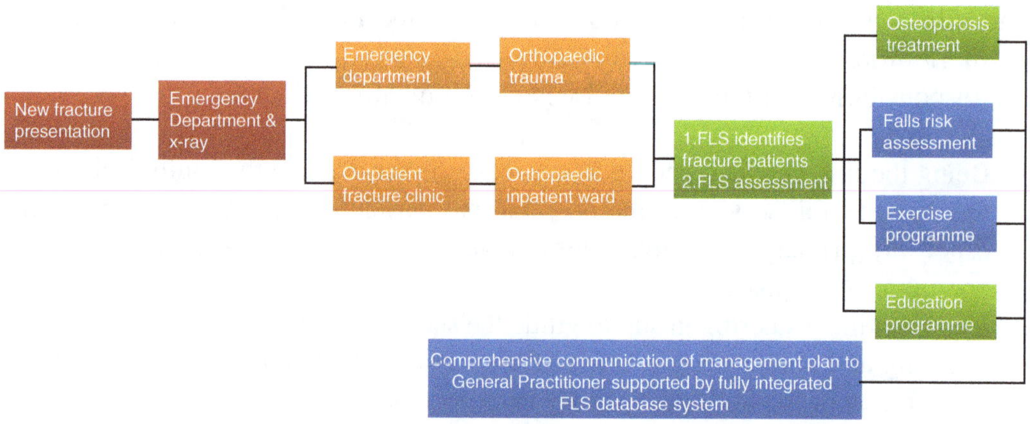

Fig. 3.1 Example of a hospital based fracture Liaison service (UK) http://capturethefracture.org/fracture-liaison-services

3.3.2 The Typical Patient Journey

Figure 3.1 provides an example of a pathway of care for people with fragility fracture using a type A model of care.

Identifying people who require the Fracture Liaison Service ('the Service') can be the most time-consuming element as this patient group is often not recorded in medical records as having sustained a 'fragility fracture' but simply a 'fracture'. Therefore, early in the development of a Service, the steering group will need to guide and support the Fracture Liaison Coordinator in the set-up of a system that makes the task less onerous but with the aim of identifying all of those requiring the Service.

International guidelines suggest that all people aged over 50 years who have a fragility fracture (whether identified through presentation with the fracture or found serendipitously through radiology for other reasons) should be assessed [30], so the identification process needs to include the following settings:

- Emergency departments (ED)—whether admitted to a ward or discharged directly from the ED
- Inpatients in all wards/units, including those who fracture while an inpatient
- Those with vertebral fractures identified on radiology reports (incidental or anticipated)
- Those referred from primary care settings but not attended ED or in a ward.

People with vertebral fractures account for about four percent of all fracture presentations and often present 'silently' and diagnosed with back pain, so special attention to finding them is required.

3.3.2.1 First Contact with People Requiring the Fracture Liaison Service

At the first meeting, an explanation of the reasons for referral to the service is required, along with a discussion about the nature of fragility fracture and osteoporosis, investigations that are required and potential results. All initial discussions should be brief, with the aim of helping the person and/or their family know why the Service is required for them. More in-depth discussions can follow later when the patient has had time to absorb the early information.

3.3.2.2 Assessment

A thorough assessment of bone health (Chap. 1) and general health status (Chap. 4) is essential. Assessment involves discussion about the mechanism of the fragility fracture, co-morbidities and the investigations needed as described in Chap. 1. Risk factors for fragility fracture are listed in Box 3.2. The probability of fracture can be estimated using a tool such as the WHO Fracture Risk Assessment Tool (FRAX®) (https://www.sheffield.ac.uk/FRAX/tool.jsp) or the Garvan fracture risk calculator (https://www.garvan.org.au/promotions/bone-fracture-risk/calculator/). While these tools should be used as a guide only and with clinical expertise on the variables that could affect scores, they can be an opportunity to help people with a fragility fracture to engage with assessment and treatment.

Box 3.2: Risk Factors for Fragility Fracture

Age Gender Low body mass index History of falls from a standing height Previous fragility fracture	Parental history of hip fracture Current glucocorticoid treatment Current smoking Alcohol intake of three or more units per day

Secondary causes of osteoporosis:
- Rheumatoid arthritis
- Type 1 diabetes
- Osteogenesis imperfecta in adults
- Long-standing untreated hyperthyroidism
- Hypogonadism/premature menopause (below 45 years)
- Chronic malnutrition
- Chronic malabsorption
- Chronic liver disease

Investigations include:

- Bone density scanning using densitometry (DXA) which has a low radiation dose in comparison to other testing mechanisms, e.g. computed tomography (CT)
- Levels of blood serum of vitamin D, calcium and, e.g. thyroid function tests and others that can suggest aetiology of osteoporosis.

3.3.2.3 Health Education

Health education is a continuing and essential strategy to be used during all interactions with a person who is accessing the Service. The aim is to support the person and their family/carer, at a pace that suits their ability to understand and respond positively. Further aims are the ability to self-manage their health-care needs, to be responsible for conservative interventions and to work effectively with their health-care team to concord with medical therapies and attend check-ups periodically to ensure their treatment remains contemporary and appropriate for them. This is also an opportunity to dispel the myths that abound about osteoporosis treatments with positive truthful explanations.

These conversations, along with formal group education, supporting the person to live well with a chronic condition, require significant skill in positively engaging the person and their family/carer, while recognising they may not be able to assimilate all information in one consultation. It is recommended that health professionals engaging in this work seek training in behaviour change strategies.

3.3.2.4 Establishing a Personal Plan

Following diagnosis, a personalised care plan needs to be set, listing agreed treatment elements and including how the person or team will work to achieve the elements, including access to services required. The person will set some goals for their self-management plan which will be reviewed at agreed timeframes to ensure the person and their health-care team are on track for success in preventing the next fracture.

3.3.2.5 Evaluation

The Fracture Liaison Coordinator is responsible for maintaining records of the progress made by people attending the Service and to share these with the team and the individual. Being able to see progress is very important in motivating them to maintain their treatment and participate in regular review when required.

3.4 Summary of Key Points

- Falls are a key cause of fragility fractures, so preventing them is an essential aspect of preventing fractures
- Holistic person-centred assessment, secondary fracture prevention and assessment and management of falls risk are essential aspects of fragility fracture care and prevention
- Risk factors for falls are individual and complex, and individual screening/assessment is an important first step in falls prevention that can lead to a fall prevention plan
- Environmental adaptations, exercise programmes, vision assessment and interventions, medication review and adjustment, footwear adjustment and foot care are important aspects of falls prevention pathways of care
- Fear of falling is a debilitating consequence of falls that requires sensitive, multidisciplinary care

- A range of system failings make it difficult and time-consuming to identify people with a fragility fracture, so there is a 'care gap' that results in many people being left undiagnosed and not treated
- Secondary fracture prevention services, known internationally as Fracture Liaison Services, aim to narrow this gap by evaluating all patients with a fragility fracture, prescribing medical and conservative care treatment that aim to improve bone density and refracture prevention and ensuring follow-up using a holistic, patient-centred multidisciplinary approach.

3.5 Further Study

- Identify the education needs of your team in relation to both falls and secondary fracture prevention and consider how these needs might be fulfilled
- Examples of education resources include:
  - IOF Capture the Fracture best practice framework http://www.capture-the-fracture.org/node/20
  - UK NOS Fracture Prevention Practitioner e-learning with test https://nos.org.uk/for-health-professionals/professional-development/e-learning-and-training/fracture-prevention-practitioner-training/
  - Local and national training programmes.

3.5.1 Self-Assessment

Assessing your own learning and performance needs to refer to both the falls and Fracture Liaison Service sections:

- Having read this chapter and undertaken further study, the following are some ideas relating to how you might identify what you have learnt and how it relates to your own practice and that of the team you work in
- Discuss the learning you have gained from this chapter and the book so far with your colleagues: identify and discuss how you, as a team, might improve local practice in prevention of falls in your unit and secondary prevention of fractures.

References

1. Ambrose A et al (2015) Falls and fractures: a systematic approach to screening and prevention. Maturitas 82:85–93
2. Curtis EM et al (2017) The impact of fragility fracture and approaches to osteoporosis risk assessment worldwide. Bone 104:29–38

3. Lippuner K et al (2008) Remaining lifetime and absolute probabilities of osteoporotic fracture in Swiss men and women. Osteoporos Int 20(7):1131–1140
4. Chipchase LS et al (2000) Hip fractures in South Australia; into the next century. ANZ J Surg 70:117–119
5. Eisman JA et al (2012) Making the first fracture the last fracture: ASBMR Task Force on Secondary Fracture Prevention. J Bone Miner Res 27(10):2039–2046
6. Bain H et al (2016) A comprehensive fracture prevention strategy in older adults: The European Union Geriatric Medicine Society (EUGMS) statement. Aging Clin Exp Res 28(4):797–803
7. Bliuc D et al (2015) Risk of subsequent fractures and mortality in elderly women and men with fragility fractures with and without osteoporotic bone density: the Dubbo Osteoporosis Epidemiology Study. J Bone Miner Res 30(4):637–646
8. Svedborn A et al (2014) Epidemiology and economic burden of osteoporosis in Switzerland. Arch Osteoporosis. 9: 187. Osteoporos Int 22(7):2051–2065
9. Ganda K et al (2013) Models of care for the secondary prevention of osteoporotic fractures: a systematic review and meta-analysis. Osteoporos Int 24(2):393–406
10. Lord SR et al (2007) Falls in older people: risk factors and strategies for prevention. Cambridge University Press, Cambridge
11. Ambrose AF et al (2013) Risk factors for fall among older adults: a review of the literature. Maturitas 75:51061
12. NICE (2013) Falls in older people: assessing risk and prevention. CG161. National Institute for Health and Care Excellence
13. Edwards N Lockett D (2008) Development and validation of a modified falls-efficacy scale. Disabil Rehabil Assist Technol 3(4):193–200
14. Podsiadlo D, Richardson S (1991) The timed "Up and Go" Test a Test of Basic Functional Mobility for Frail Elderly Persons. J Am Geriatr Soc 39:142–148
15. Hoffheinz M, Mibs MPH (2016) The prognostic validity of the timed up and go test with a dual tasks for predicting the risk of falls in the elderly. Gerontol Geriatr Med 2:1–5
16. Tinetti M et al (1990) Falls Efficacy as a Measure of Fear or Falling. J Gerontol 45:239
17. Tinetti ME et al (1986) Fall Risk Index for elderly patients based on number of chronic disabilities. Am J Med 80:429–434
18. Stevens J et al (2014) Circumstances and outcomes of falls among high risk community-dwelling older adults. Injury Epidemiol 1:5
19. Gillespie LD et al (2012) Interventions for preventing falls in older people living in the community. Cochrane Database Syst Rev 2012;(9):CD007146
20. Kendrick D et al (2014) Exercise for reducing fear of falling in older people living in the community. Cochrane Database Syst Rev 11:CD009848
21. Karlsson MK et al (2013) Prevention of falls in the elderly—a review. Osteoporos Int 24(3):747–762
22. Reed-Jones R et al (2013) Vision and falls: a multidisciplinary review of the contributions of visual impairment to falls among older adults. Muturitas 75:22–28
23. Huang AR et al (2013) Medication-related falls in the elderly. Causative factors and preventive strategies. Drugs Aging 29(5):359–376
24. Spink MJ et al (2011) Effectiveness of a multifaceted podiatry intervention to prevent falls in community dwelling older people with disabling foot pain: randomized controlled trial. BMJ 342:d3411
25. Kelsey JL et al (2010) Footwear and falls in the home among older individuals in the MOBILIZE Boston study. Footwear Sci 2(3):123–129
26. Parry S (2013) How should we manage fear of falling on older adults living the community? BMJ 346:f2933
27. Nakayama A et al (2016) Evidence of effectiveness of a fracture liaison service to reduce the re-fracture rate. Osteoporos Int 27(3):873–879

28. Akesson K et al (2013) Capture the fracture: a Best Practice Framework and global campaign to break the fragility fracture cycle. Osteoporos Int 24:2135–2152
29. Marsh D et al (2011) Coordinator-based systems for secondary prevention of fragility fractures. Osteoporos Int 22:2051–2065
30. NOS (National Osteoporosis Society) (2016) Competency framework for fracture prevention practitioners https://nos.org.uk/for-health-professionals/tools-resources/

4 Comprehensive Geriatric Assessment from a Nursing Perspective

Lina Spirgiene and Louise Brent

As the incidence of fragility fractures continues to rise, healthcare professionals will encounter patients with fractures in a variety of clinical settings such as falls clinics, intermediate care services and acute medical wards. Older people with fragility fractures are a diverse group, and their care needs are complex. Although some have comparatively few health problems, many have a series of interconnected illnesses and psychological and social problems requiring a range of therapeutic interventions. The primary focus of care is to meet the needs of the older person following skeletal trauma throughout their care pathway and ensure that they receive the same high standard of specialist care within orthopaedic services as they would within a setting specialising in the care of older people. The central philosophy should be holistic care using a person-centred approach that brings the various aspects of specialist care together.

'Geriatric syndrome' is a term often used to refer to common health problems in older adults that do not fit into distinct organ-specific disease categories and that have multifactorial causes; this includes problems such as frailty, cognitive impairment, delirium, incontinence, malnutrition, falls, gait disorders, pressure ulcers, sleep disorders, sensory deficits, fatigue and dizziness. These are common in older adults and can have a major impact on quality of life (QoL) and disability [1]. Geriatric syndromes can best be identified by a comprehensive multidisciplinary

L. Spirgiene, R.N., Ph.D. (✉)
Medical Academy, Faculty of Nursing, Department of Nursing and Care, Lithuanian University of Health Sciences, Kaunas, Lithuania

Nursing Coordination Department, Hospital of Lithuanian University of Health Sciences Kauno Klinikos, Kaunas, Lithuania

L. Brent
National Office of Clinical Audit, St Stephen's Green, Dublin 2, Ireland
e-mail: louisebrent@noca.ie

K. Hertz, J. Santy-Tomlinson (eds.), *Fragility Fracture Nursing*, Perspectives in Nursing Management and Care for Older Adults, https://doi.org/10.1007/978-3-319-76681-2_4

geriatric assessment so that they can inform planning appropriate interventions within a team approach.

Problems that relate to ageing such as functional impairment and dementia are common and often unrecognised or inadequately addressed. Identifying problems specific to ageing so that interventions can be tailored to meet the specific needs of patients with fragility fractures requires a detailed and comprehensive assessment that can help clinicians manage these conditions and prevent or delay their complications. This needs to be conducted by the whole multidisciplinary team so that the skills of each team member can contribute to building a picture of the patient's needs. Nursing assessment is a significant part of this whole. A term often used in relation to the assessment of older people with medical needs is *comprehensive geriatric assessment* (CGA). This approach is designed to accommodate the multidisciplinary approach that is so important in the care of the older person in any setting, and the role of nursing assessment within this is central to planning effective interventions to resolve nursing-focused problems.

The aim of this chapter is to explore the nature of comprehensive geriatric assessment (CGA) for the patient with a fragility fracture and discuss how this can be applied to nursing assessment and care.

4.1 Learning Outcomes

At the end of the chapter, and following further study, the nurse will be able to:

- Explain the principles of comprehensive geriatric assessment (CGA) from a nursing perspective
- Identify how the CGA process applies to the whole multidisciplinary team
- Discuss the nursing contribution to comprehensive assessment of the older person with fragility fracture.

4.2 The Concept of CGA

Assessment involves collecting information about a person's circumstances and needs and making sense of that information to help in decision-making about what support, treatment and care is needed; it should be timely and comprehensive [2]. The assessment of older people differs from standard medical review in three ways: (1) it focuses on older people with complex problems; (2) it emphasises functional status and quality of life; and (3) it takes advantage of an interdisciplinary team. Getting to know people, their strengths and needs is an important first step in effective care of older people [3], and this has been reflected in the APIE (assessment, planning, implementation and evaluation) approach to nursing for more than 50 years. It is recognised that older people receiving nursing care should have the same comprehensive assessment and risk identification to facilitate the identification of individual needs, care planning and identification of risks that might impact on optimal care outcomes and inform effective discharge planning [4].

Comprehensive geriatric assessment (CGA) is a multidimensional, interdisciplinary process designed to detect and assess frailty [5], to determine a frail older person's medical conditions, mental health, functional capacity and social circumstances [6] and to identify their care and treatment needs. There is strong evidence that CGA can reduce mortality, increase the number of patients who can return home after hospitalisation and reduce length of stay [7]. The purpose is to plan and carry out a holistic plan for treatment, rehabilitation, support and long-term follow-up [8]. CGA is part of an integrated approach to assessment based on the following principles [9]:

- The process is person-centred
- The older person's capacity to participate in the process voluntarily must be assessed; if capacity does not exist, there should be a system in place that considers their needs within an ethical framework
- Links between social and healthcare need to be made so that older people who need CGA receive it efficiently in a way that considers their degree of need in timely manner
- Assessments are carried out to a reliable standard within and across multidisciplinary teams.

Models of CGA have evolved in different healthcare settings and to meet differing needs, although not specifically in relation to the management of the patient with fragility fracture. The skill, at the heart of orthogeriatric care, when working with patients with fragility fracture is developing a comprehensive picture of the potential impact of co-morbidities and functional capacity to try to predict their potential impact on the patient's recovery and rehabilitation following the fracture [6] and for this knowledge to direct healthcare practice. There is limited discussion of the role of nurses in the process of CGA as its development has been led by geriatricians. There is good reason, however, for nurses to begin to incorporate CGA into their own practice with patients with fragility fractures because of its potential to provide a clear overview of the patient's healthcare and nursing needs. This may mean that nurses will need to adapt the process to reflect the purpose of nursing and to avoid an overly medicalised approach to care.

Common to CGA are several key features that have been attributed with its effectiveness and can be applied to the patient with fragility fracture, including [10]:

- Co-ordinated multidisciplinary assessment, so that each member of the team can contribute expertise; the team is commonly made up of a geriatrician/physician, nurse and therapists but can involve other health professionals depending on need
- One team member 'in charge' as the co-ordinator or 'case manager' of the process
- Geriatric medicine expertise, so that the medical management of the patient's health problems can lead multidisciplinary interventions

- Identification of medical, physical, social and psychological problems, so that a comprehensive picture can be obtained and the impact of each of these understood
- Leading to the formation of a plan of care that includes appropriate rehabilitation.

The first step in CGA is to identify those individuals who are likely to benefit from this process as well as the orthogeriatric team approach. Decision-making criteria used to identify patients could include:

- The age of the person and the way in which their ageing process is manifested, e.g. frailty
- Existing medical conditions that are likely to impact on care, recovery and outcomes
- The presence of psychosocial disorders such as depression or social isolation
- Specific 'geriatric syndrome' conditions such as dementia, falls, functional disability, sarcopenia and frailty
- Previous or predicted high need for healthcare use
- Recent change in living situation, e.g. from independent living to assisted living, nursing home or in-home caregivers
- Major illnesses such as those requiring hospitalisation (such as a fracture) or increased need for home care resources to manage medical and functional needs.

The CGA process should begin on admission, encompassing emergency care; but it is not a one-off process, so should continue throughout the care process with constant review and evaluation. To facilitate recording and sharing of assessment findings, the multidisciplinary team should share documentation that includes a pro-forma to help clinicians to follow the process. In an ideal world, the same process should follow the older person after discharge to home care and other community-based care facilities.

Performing a comprehensive assessment is an ambitious undertaking and is often more complex than it may seem (Box 4.1), as older people often struggle to recall their past medical history and cognitive impairment can make it difficult for them to answer questions. Resolving this issue involves skilled communication with the patient and collaboration with family and other people who know the patient well to help with history taking.

Box 4.1: Areas of Assessment That Team Members May Choose to Assess Depending on Patient Needs

- Current symptoms and illnesses and their functional impact
- Current medications, their indications and effects
- Relevant past illnesses

- Recent and impending life changes
- Objective measure of overall personal and social functionality
- Current and future living environment and its appropriateness to function and prognosis
- Family situation and availability
- Current caregiver network including its deficiencies and potential
- Objective measure of cognitive status
- Objective assessment of mobility and balance
- Rehabilitative status and prognosis if ill or disabled
- Current emotional health and substance abuse
- Nutritional status and needs
- Disease risk factors, screening status and health promotion activities
- Services required and received

Conceptually, CGA involves several processes of care that are shared over several members of the assessment team (Box 4.2).

Box 4.2: Elements of Comprehensive Geriatric Care

- Data gathering
- Biopsychosocial assessment
- Discussions among the team
- Patient and/or caregiver as a member of the team involvement
- Treatment and nursing plan development, with the patient and/or caregiver
- Implementation of the treatment and nursing plan
- Monitoring response to the treatment and nursing plan
- Revising the treatment and nursing plan

CGA, undertaken by multiple personnel over many encounters, is best suited for older people with multiple medical problems and significant functional limitations. An interdisciplinary team, representing medicine, psychiatry, social work, nutrition, physical and occupational therapy and others, should perform a shared detailed assessment, analyse the information, devise a collaborative intervention strategy, initiate treatment and follow up on the patient's progress.

Significantly, older patients are likely to survive admission to hospital and return home if they undergo CGA, while they are inpatients [11], and, if indicated, it should be initiated as soon as possible after admission by a skilled, senior member of the multidisciplinary team and used to identify reversible medical problems, target rehabilitation goals and plan all the components of discharge and post-discharge support needs [12].

4.3 Dimensions of Comprehensive Geriatric Assessment

Comprehensive assessment involves looking not only at disease states as a standard medical assessment would do, or at functional ability as a standard rehabilitation assessment might do, but at a range of domains. By assessing each of these domains of health, a comprehensive assessment can be made, and the full biopsychosocial nature of the individual's problems can be identified. This process can be supported by using standardised scales and tools, or full formal assessment schemes such as the 'interrai' assessment tools (www.interrai.org). Using standardised scales can encourage consistent practice, help to ensure safety (e.g. pressure injury risk screening) and enable detection of serial changes, but they can also be time-consuming and clinically constraining. Clinicians undertaking CGA should consider the extent to which standardised approaches are helpful in their setting [12]. Core components of CGA that should be considered during the assessment process are outlined in Table 4.1.

Functional status: Functional status relates to the ability to perform activities necessary or desirable in daily life. It is directly influenced by health conditions, particularly in the context of an older person's environment and social support network. Changes in functional status (e.g. not being able to bathe independently) should prompt further diagnostic evaluation and intervention. Measurement of

Table 4.1 Domains and suggested items for comprehensive geriatric assessment (BGS 2010)

Domain	Suggested items for assessment
Physical health and medical conditions	Comorbid conditions and disease severity Medical review Nutritional status Polypharmacy Urinary continence Sexual function Vision/hearing Dentition
Mental health and psychological status	Cognition Mood and anxiety Fears Goals of care Advance care preferences Spirituality
Functioning	Functional capacity: core functions such as mobility and balance, fall risk Activities of daily living Life roles that are important to the patient
Social circumstances	Social support and networks: Informal support available from family Wider network of friends and contacts Statutory care Financial concerns and poverty
Environment	Living situation: housing, comfort, facilities and safety Use or potential use of 'telehealth' technology Transport facilities Accessibility to local resources

functional status can be valuable in monitoring response to treatment and can provide prognostic information that assists in long-term care planning. With respect to the impact of functional status on activities of daily living (ADLs), an older person's functional status can be assessed at three levels: (1) basic activities of daily living (BADLs), (2) instrumental or intermediate activities of daily living (IADLs) and (3) advanced activities of daily living (AADLs). BADLs consider self-care tasks which include; bathing, dressing, toileting and maintaining continence, grooming, feeding and transferring. IADLs consider the ability to maintain an independent household which includes shopping for groceries, driving or using public transportation, using the telephone, performing housework, home maintenance, preparing meals, doing laundry, taking medication and handling finances.

In addition to considering ADLs, gait speed alone predicts functional decline and early mortality in older adults. Assessment of gait speed is the domain of the physiotherapist within the team and may identify patients who need further evaluation, such as those at increased risk of falls. Assessing gait speed may also help identify frail patients who might not benefit from treatment of chronic asymptomatic diseases such as hypertension. For example, elevated blood pressure in individuals age 65 and older is associated with increased mortality only in individuals with a walking speed ≥0.8 m/s (measured over 6 m or 20 feet) [13].

Falls: Approximately one-third of community-dwelling people over 65 years and one-half of those over 80 years of age fall each year [14]. Those who have fallen or have a gait or balance problem are at higher risk of having a subsequent fall and losing independence. An assessment of fall risk should be integrated into the history and physical examination of all older patients (Chap. 3).

Cognition: The incidence of dementia and delirium increase with age, particularly among those over 85 years; yet many older people with cognitive impairment remain undiagnosed. The value of making an early diagnosis includes the possibility of uncovering treatable conditions. The evaluation of cognitive function can include a thorough history, brief cognition screening, a detailed mental status examination, neuropsychological testing and other tests to evaluate medical conditions that may contribute to cognitive impairment (Chap. 9).

Mood: Depressive illness in older people is a serious health concern leading to unnecessary suffering, impaired functional status, increased mortality and excessive use of healthcare resources (Chap. 9). Depression in later life remains underdiagnosed and inadequately treated. Depression in older adults may present atypically and may be masked in patients with cognitive impairment. Screening is easily administered and likely to identify patients at risk if both of the folowing questions are answered affirmatively:

1. 'During the past month, have you been bothered by feeling down, depressed, or hopeless?'
2. 'During the past month, have you been bothered by little interest or pleasure in doing things?'

Polypharmacy: Older people are often prescribed multiple medications by different healthcare providers, placing them at increased risk of drug interactions and adverse medication events. The clinician should review medications at each visit. The best method of detecting potential problems with polypharmacy is to have patients provide all medications (prescription and non-prescription) in their packaging. Alternatively, practitioners should contact the patient's primary care physician, particularly if the patient cannot remember their medications. As some health systems have moved towards electronic health records and electronic prescribing, the possibility of detecting potential medication errors and interactions has increased. Older people should also be asked about alternative medical therapies by asking about herbal medicine use with the question: 'What prescription medications, over the counter medicines, vitamins, herbs, or supplements do you use?'

Social and financial support: The existence of a strong social support network in an older person's life can frequently be the determining factor of whether the patient can remain at home or needs placement in a residential care setting. A brief screen of social support includes taking a social history and determining who would be available to help if they become ill. Early identification of problems with social support can help planning and timely development of resource referrals. For patients with functional impairment, the practitioner should ascertain who the person has available to help with ADLs. It is also important to assess the financial situation of a functionally impaired older adult; some may qualify for state or local benefits, depending upon their income. Occasionally, there are other benefits such as long-term care insurance or veteran's benefits that can help in paying for caregivers and prevent the need for institutionalisation.

The gathering of information is more complex than it seems [7], particularly collecting accurate baseline information from patients who may have cognitive difficulties, espeically if the environment is noisy such as in the ED or busy trauma unit, in the presence of pain or opioid analgesia use or anaesthesia. In the first few hours following admission, the patient is more likely to recall the history of the injury due to more recent recall, but this period is also very stressful. Collecting detailed and accurate information needs specialised skills in communication and an expert understanding of the process of assessment.

4.4 Assessment Tools

Although the amount of potentially important information may seem overwhelming, formal assessment tools and shortcuts can reduce this burden on the clinician performing the initial CGA. A previsit questionnaire sent to the patient or caregiver prior to the initial assessment can be timesaving when there is a need to gather a large amount of information and timing allows, although this is rarely an option when there is an acute admission. Questionnaires can be used to gather information about general history (e.g. past medical history, medications, social history, review of systems), as well as gather information specific to CGA, such as:

- Ability to perform functional tasks and need for assistance
- Fall history
- Urinary and/or faecal incontinence

- Pain
- Sources of social support, particularly family or friends
- Depressive symptoms
- Vision or hearing difficulties
- Whether the patient has specified a 'lasting power of attorney' for healthcare.

Support staff can be trained to administer screening instruments to both save time and help the clinician to focus on specific disabilities that need more detailed evaluation.

4.5 Posthospital Discharge

Key elements of posthospital discharge CGA include targeting criteria to identify vulnerable patients, a programme of multidimensional assessment, comprehensive discharge planning and home follow-up by nurses with specialised geriatric practitioner training who visit patients during hospitalisation and at least twice during the weeks following discharge. This intervention is usually initiated 1–2 days prior to hospital discharge. Like home assessments, post-discharge home visits are supplemented by telephone calls and additional visits by physical therapy, occupational therapy, social work and/or home nursing services when indicated (Chap. 10).

4.6 Secondary Prevention

Secondary prevention of fragility fractures (Chap. 3) should be approached in a systematic and coordinated manner, to some extent during the inpatient stay, but continuing after discharge. All patients presenting with fragility fractures should be assessed by an orthogeriatrician or other specialist with respect to their ongoing fracture risk. This may trigger referral to other specialists such as endocrinologists for further investigation. Referrals must also be made to secondary fracture prevention services (Chap. 3) where patients can be reviewed by a fracture prevention practitioner, orthogeriatrician, endocrinologist and dietician. The assessment, diagnosis and referral process can be coordinated by a fracture prevention practitioner and treatment initiated and followed up accordingly. Patients should also be referred, where appropriate, to falls clinics.

4.7 The CGA Team

The assessment team varies depending on the service and can include the full range of healthcare professionals working in the multidisciplinary team. In many settings, the CGA process relies on a core team consisting of a medical clinician, nurse, therapist and social worker and, when appropriate, draws upon an extended team including occupational and other therapists, nutritionists, pharmacists, psychiatrists, psychologists, dentists, audiologists, podiatrists and ophthalmologists/optometrists.

Although these professionals can work in the hospital setting, many are also available in the community. Increasingly, there is a move towards a 'virtual team' concept in which members are included as needed, assessments are conducted at different locations on different days, often using the electronic health record but stored electronically and accessible anywhere, and team communication is completed via telephone or electronically,.

Traditionally, the various components of the process are completed by different members of the team, with considerable variability in the way assessments are conducted and recorded. The medical assessment of older people may be conducted by a physician (usually a geriatrician), nurse practitioner, physiotherapist or physician assistant. The core team (geriatrician, nurse, therapist, social worker) may conduct only brief initial assessments or screening for some dimensions. These may be subsequently augmented with more in-depth assessments by additional professionals; e.g. a dietitian may be needed to assess dietary intake and make recommendations on optimising nutrition, or an audiologist may need to conduct a more extensive assessment of hearing loss and evaluate an older person for a hearing aid.

Because of the 24-h nature of their practice and the wide range of care, nurses are often expected to take a leading role in the care of older people and to coordinate the assessment process. Despite this, the role of the nurse in CGA is ill defined and is not considered in detail in the literature. The potential for nurses, particularly those with advanced assessment skills, to act as a fulcrum for the CGA process is largely untapped. Nursing is already directed by the nursing process: incorporating APIE. Clarke [3] suggests that this traditional view of the nursing process focuses on identifying need deficit and that a more effective philosophy is to assess the resources of older people themselves and jointly plan care alongside the MDT, patients and carers so that as much self-management is retained as possible. Nurses place importance on coming to know a person as an individual through a continuous and ongoing assessment process that will support the rest of the nursing process (planning, implementation and evaluation) and help them to provide effective care. This knowledge can only be achieved by a comprehensive assessment process that incorporates the biological, psychological, social and spiritual dimensions of the person [15].

While the CGA process has not been specifically developed to capture patients' nursing needs, it has the potential to become a holistic multidisciplinary assessment for the whole team and to ensure that the complex needs of patients with fragility fractures are fully met through a continuous process while looking for changes in the patient's condition. The whole team need to work together to further develop this process from a collaborative perspective so that the many different forms of mono-disciplinary assessment processes and associated documentation can be brought together as a single, effective process [4]. New or adapted assessment tools may be required for use by all professionals in the team that can be used to facilitate multidisciplinary and interagency working [16] but also with a view to seamless transfers between primary and secondary care settings. All practitioners should be able to use the information generated during CGA to develop treatment and long-term follow-up plans, arrange for primary care and rehabilitative services, organise and facilitate the intricate process of case management, determine long-term care requirements and optimal placement and make the best use of healthcare resources.

The assessment process in most units is not perfect, and there is a need to identify ways to both improve the assessment process and demonstrate the value of nursing in this central aspect of care.

4.8 Summary of Key Points

- Timely and comprehensive assessment is essential in understanding the needs of older people and ensuring that their needs are met through care and treatment
- CGA is a person-centred, holistic, multidisciplinary process that helps to assess the frail older person so that their medical conditions, mental health, functional capacity and social circumstances can be considered in detail and from which patients with fragility fractures can benefit significantly
- The process should begin on admission and be followed through to post-discharge care in primary and residential care settings: it is not a one-off process but should be subjected to constant review and evaluation
- The CGA process should, as a minimum, consider the domains of physical health and medical conditions, mental health and psychological status, functioning, social circumstances and environment so that MDT care and treatment can be based on the needs generated by these
- Assessment tools need to be developed, or adapted, to meet the needs of this interdisciplinary process and can include existing assessment and screening tools. Interdisciplinary team collaboration will be needed in making this process work in the best interests of patients with fragility fractures.

4.9 Suggested Further Study

- Think about how you currently conduct assessment in your place of work—does it fit in with the CGA approach to assessment?
- What skills do you/your team need for you to improve how you assess patients using this approach?
- How might you learn these skills and how would you assess what you have learnt?
- Discuss with other members of the multidisciplinary team within which you work how you might move towards a full team approach to the CGA process and what changes might be needed for this to happen.

4.10 Self-Assessment

- Examine the current assessment documentation used in your unit and consider whether it reflects:
  - Comprehensiveness
  - Patient-centeredness
  - Multidisciplinary team working
- Reflect on how this could be adapted and improved.

References

1. Inouye SK et al (2007) Geriatric syndromes: clinical, research and policy implications of a core geriatric concept. J Am Geriatr Soc 55(5):780–791
2. Slater P, McCormack B (2005) Determining older people's needs for care by Registered Nurses: the Nursing Needs Assessment Tool. J Adv Nurs 52(6):601–608
3. Clarke CL (2012) Fundamentals of nursing. In: Reed J et al (eds) Nursing older adults. Open University Press, Maidenhead, pp 79–79
4. Langdon R et al (2013) Assessment of the elderly: it's worth covering the risks. J Nurs Manag 21:94–105
5. Smith G, Kydd A (2016) Editorial: Getting care of older people right. The need for appropriate frailty assessment. J Clin Nurs 26:5–6
6. British Geriatric Society (BGS), Comprehensive assessment of the frail older patient. 2010. http://www.bgs.org.uk/good-practice-guides/resources/goodpractice/gpgcgassessment#
7. Wilson, H. (2017) Pre-operative management. In: Falaschi, P. & Marsh, D. Orthogeriatrics. Springer: Basel pp 63-79
8. Stuck AE et al (1993) Comprehensive geriatric assessment: a meta-analysis of controlled trials. Lancet 342:1032
9. Devons CA (2002) Comprehensive geriatric assessment: making the most of the aging years. Curr Opin Clin Nutr Metab Care 5:19
10. Ellis G et al (2011) Comprehensive geriatric assessment for older adults admitted to hospital: meta-analysis of randomised controlled trials. BMJ 343:d6553
11. Oliver D et al (2014) Making our health and care systems fit for an ageing population. Kings Fund, London
12. Welsh TJ et al (2014) Comprehensive geriatric assessment—a guide for the non-specialist. Int J Clin Pract 68(3):290–293
13. Studenski S et al (2011) Gait speed and survival in older adults. JAMA 305(1):0–58
14. Lord SR et al (2007) Falls in older people: risk factors and strategies for prevention. Cambridge University Press, Cambridge
15. Locsin RC, Purnell MJ (2009) A contemporary nursing process. Springer, New York
16. Folder-Like et al (2013) Development and evidence base of a new efficient assessment instrument for international use by nurses in community settings with older people. Int J Nurs Stud 50:1180–1183

5 Orthogeriatric Nursing in the Emergency and Perioperative In-Patient Setting

Charlotte Myhre Jensen, Karen Hertz, and Oliver Mauthner

As the population ages, musculoskeletal trauma in older people will be a growing challenge. Although management of older people following trauma has some similarities to that for all trauma, there are also differences and specific considerations relating to ageing. The most common cause of injury in older people is a fall, so fall-related trauma will be the focus of this section while acknowledging that the care of elderly trauma, whatever the cause, is based on the same principles.

The aim of this chapter is to outline the care of older people with fragility fractures of the hip, the most significant injury requiring orthogeriatric care. Although the chapter is concerned with nursing interventions in orthogeriatric care generally, hip fracture is the most common reason for admission to an orthopaedic unit and the complexity of needs, prevalence, number of bed days and cost means that the focus of care tends to be predominantly on this category of injury. The principal skills and knowledge needed to look after patients with hip fractures well apply across the management of all older people with fractures and includes all the fundamental aspects of nursing care for the adult as well as specialised interventions for older people [1, 2].

C. M. Jensen, M.Ed., R.N. (✉)
Department of Orthopaedic Surgery and Traumatology, Odense University Hospital, Odense, Denmark
e-mail: Charlotte.myhre.jensen@rsyd.dk

K. Hertz (✉)
Specialised Division, University Hospital of North Midlands, Stoke-on Trent, Staffordshire, UK
e-mail: Karen.hertz@uhnm.nhs.uk

O. Mauthner, Ph.D.
Felix Platter—Spital, Basel, Switzerland

University of Basel, Basel, Switzerland
e-mail: Oliver.mauthner@unibas.ch

K. Hertz, J. Santy-Tomlinson (eds.), *Fragility Fracture Nursing*, Perspectives in Nursing Management and Care for Older Adults, https://doi.org/10.1007/978-3-319-76681-2_5

5.1 Learning Outcomes

At the end of the chapter, and following further study, the nurse will be able to:

- Identify crucial factors that impact on the outcomes of hip fracture
- Explain hip fracture types and their management
- Deliver evidence-based acute and perioperative care to patients with hip fracture
- Maintain safety and prevent and recognise complications
- Comprehensively prepare for patient discharge.

5.2 Perioperative Care

Surgery is the preferred treatment for hip fracture because it provides stable fixation, facilitates full weight bearing and decreases the risk of complications [3]. Conservative management carries additional risks of immobility, thromboembolism, pressure injuries, other complications and loss of independence. There are three phases to perioperative care: preoperative, intraoperative and postoperative.

The preoperative phase is the period prior to arrival in the operating department for surgery. The goals are to stabilise the injury, manage pain and restore function, and standardised preoperative assessments and patient-centred management protocols are needed. The aim is to facilitate prompt preparation for surgery through coordinated orthogeriatric and anesthetic care.

Intraoperative care aims to mitigate the pathophysiological effects of surgery without destabilising the patient's physiology. Patients are at substantial risk of perioperative morbidity and mortality due to age and frailty, so they have decreased physiological reserve; one or more comorbidities, polypharmacy and cognitive dysfunction are common and can have a negative impact on physiology.

Postoperatively, orthogeriatric care aims to mitigate the effects of surgery and remobilise, re-enable and remotivate patients in preparation for discharge, ideally back to their place of residence before the fracture. The early postoperative phase is crucial, as delayed remobilisation is associated with prolonged hosptial stay [4]. Postoperative care includes, therefore, early mobilisation, pain management, postoperative hypotension and fluid management, postsurgical anemia management, delirium assessment and nutritional optimisation.

5.3 Preoperative Care

Sustaining a hip fracture is a sudden traumatic event, threatening many aspects of patients' lives and a forceful reminder of their mortality [5, 6]. Factors affecting outcomes following hip fracture are dominated by restoring function, so physical care attracts the most attention. The primary goal of nursing care for the older adult with fragility hip fracture is to maximise mobility and preserve optimal function [1, 2]; psychosocial factors, however, must be incorporated into a holistic approach to care so that patients can be motivated to rehabilitate [1, 5]. Assessment and subsequent care is best provided by effective multidisciplinary team working based on sound "orthogeriatric" principles; treating the fracture while considering the causes and effects of the fall and the unstable comorbidities and initiating effective rehabilitation while considering bone health with the aim of preventing further fractures.

Emergency departments (EDs) are noisy, busy, overstimulating places, making them inappropriate care environments for vulnerable older people in a state of personal and physical crisis. Avoiding the impact of this situation requires consideration of the following three principles [7]:

- *Timeliness*—avoiding unnecessary and unwanted delay
- *Effectiveness*—aiming for optimal outcomes using the best available evidence
- *Patient-centeredness*—care that is respectful of and responsive to individual needs.

Providing care to older people following trauma must follow the same principles as for all age groups, using the ABCDE approach. The normal and abnormal changes of ageing, compounded by active comorbidities, mean that morbidity and mortality are increased concerns. Examples of physiological considerations relating to ageing include:

Airway—ageing causes degeneration of the physiological airway and musculoskeletal pathology, such as osteoarthritis, can reduce neck and spine flexibility, making airway management difficult.

Breathing—loss of respiratory resilience means loss of hypoxic reserve and potential hypoventilation with oxygen administration; oxygen therapy is still needed but requires closer monitoring in recognition of this. Older people are more at risk of respiratory failure because of the increased work of breathing.

Circulation—reduction in cardiopulmonary reserve means that there is increased risk of fluid overload when administering intravenous fluids (particularly colloids), requiring closer monitoring. Normal heart rate and blood pressure are not a guarantee of normal cardiac output and use of beta-blockers and antihypertensive agents can mask the signs of deterioration. Blood loss from the fracture site can vary from a few millilitres for an undisplaced intracapsular fracture to over a litre for a multi-fragment or subtrochanteric fracture. All patients should have intravenous saline from the time of presentation, with the rate of infusion adjusted according to the estimated blood loss and degree of dehydration.

Disability—prolonged inactivity and disuse limits ultimate functional outcome and impacts on survival.

Exposure—skin and connective tissue undergo extensive changes with ageing, resulting in diminished thermoregulation, increased risk of infection, poor wound healing and increased susceptibility to hypothermia.

A full and comprehensive history should include relevant comorbidities and medication history and previous functional ability as well as personal and social history. Many older people, with and without cognitive impairment, are unable to provide an accurate history, so the history should also be sought from a relative, caregiver or general practitioner [8]. Patients' skin should also be thoroughly examined to identify skin problems and potential skin breakdown. To prevent pressure injuries, patients should be transferred to a bed with a pressure-relieving/redistributing mattress as soon as possible (Chap. 7).

5.4 Hip Fracture Diagnosis and Surgery

A hip fracture is diagnosed by the symptoms and verified with X-rays [9]; these may be supplemented with MRI or CT to establish diagnosis. Most hip fractures occur in one of two locations; at the femoral neck or in the intertrochanteric region. The location of the fracture and the degree of displacement or impaction help determine the best treatment (Fig. 5.1). In nearly all cases, surgery is the treatment of choice as this is the most effective way to manage pain and stabilise the fracture so that the patient can remobilise as soon as possible.

Femoral neck fracture: This occurs in the neck region of the femur in the intracapsular region (within the hip joint capsule). The blood supply to this area means that, if displaced, this type of fracture may disrupt the blood supply to the femoral head, causing it to collapse due to necrosis. Hence, if the fracture is displaced, it is usually

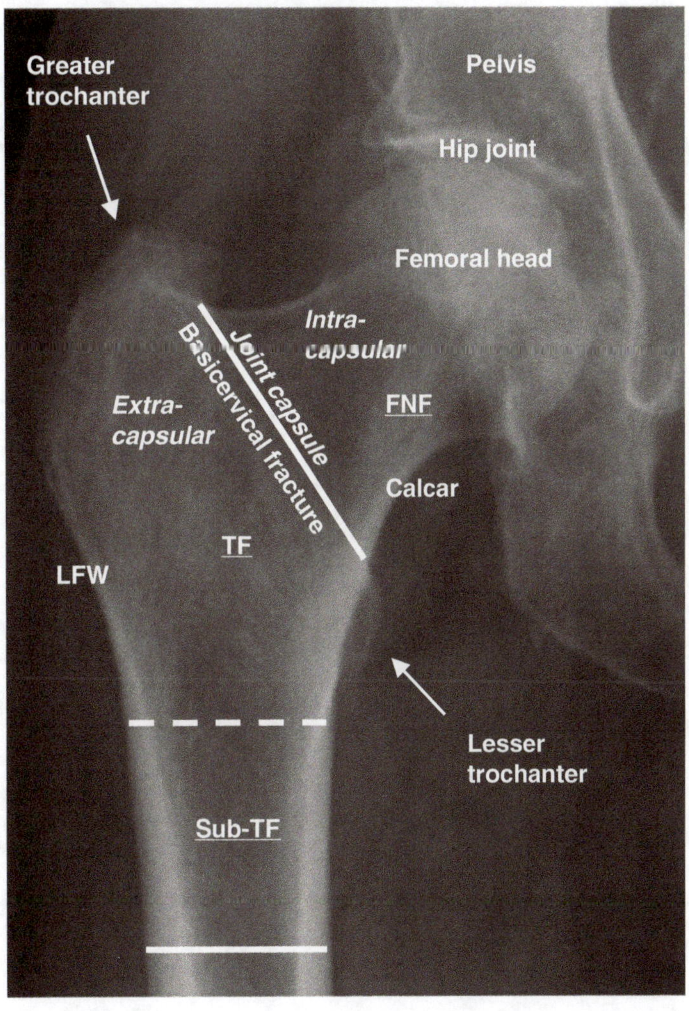

Fig. 5.1 Anteroposterior radiograph of the right side of the proximal femur showing anatomy and fracture positions. *FNF* femoral neck fracture; *TF* trochanteric fracture; *Sub-TF* subtrochanteric fracture; *LFW* lateral femoral wall (From Palm 2017 [4] with permission)

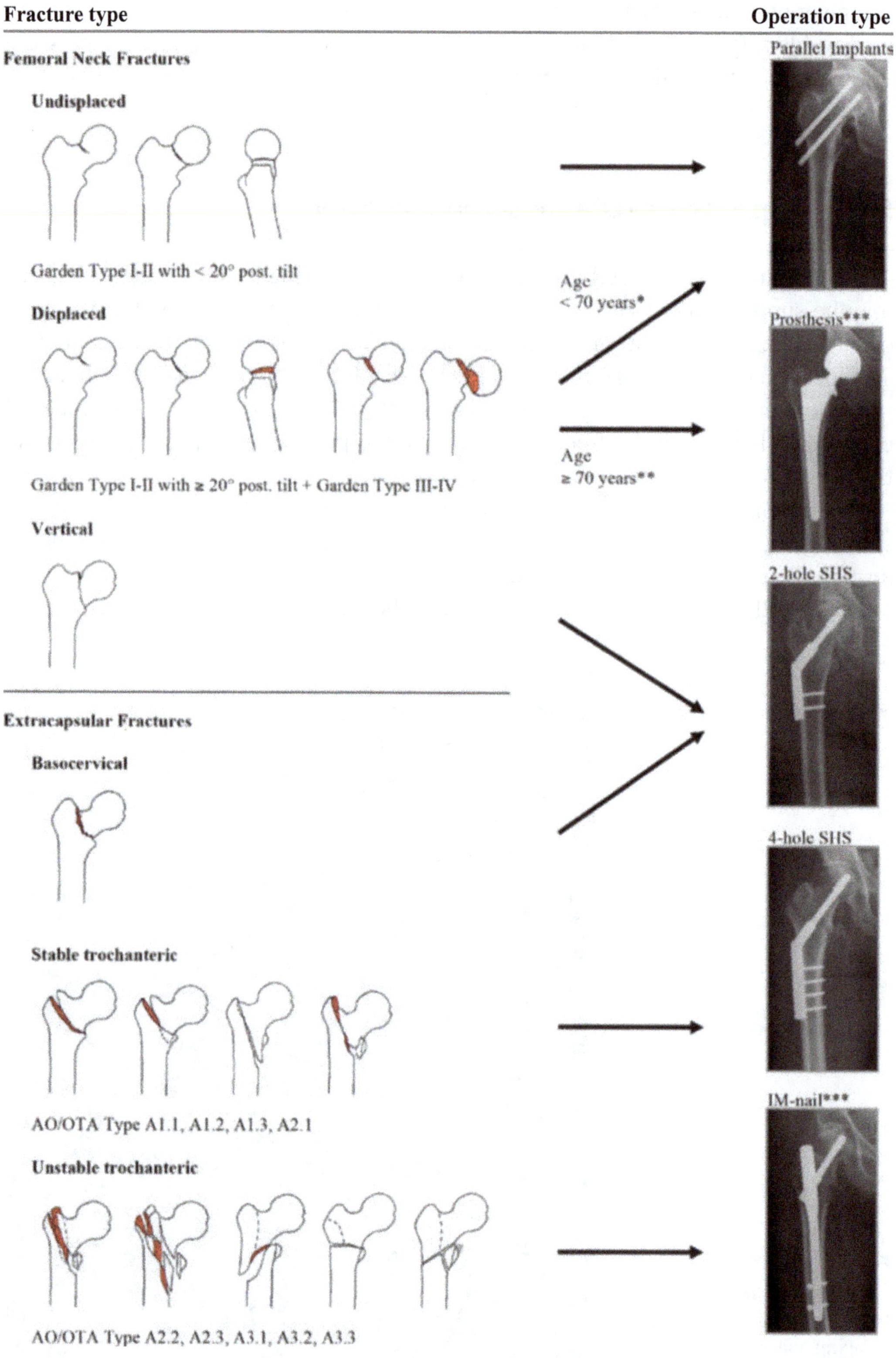

*Prosthesis, if not fully reducible on traction table. **Femoral head removal, if no pre-fracture mobility. ***Mandatory supervision of junior residents. SHS: Sliding hips screw. IM-nail: Intramedullary nail.

Fig. 5.2 How hip fracture surgery decisions are made: an algorithm for hip fracture surgery (Reproduced with permission from *Acta Orthop*)

managed with hemi-arthroplasty. Undisplaced fractures are managed with parallel implants.

Intertrochanteric hip fracture: An intertrochanteric hip fracture occurs in the upper 8–12 cm of the femoral shaft in the region between the lesser and greater trochanters. As an extracapsular fracture (outside the joint capsule), the blood supply is less likely to be disrupted, so internal fixation can be performed with nails, screws, and/or plates (see Figs. 5.1 and 5.2).

Caring for patients following hip fracture is an everyday event for care staff, but, for the patient, it is a life-changing event with severe and frightening consequences [10, 11]. Although management usually follows standardised guidelines, each person needs holistic and individual care. The aim of preoperative care is to prepare the patient for surgery in a manner that avoids the development of complications of immobility and surgery.

5.5 Pain Management

A hip fracture is very painful, but good pain management is a frequently ignored aspect of care and pain may contribute to worse outcomes. One significant reason for inadequate analgesia is poor assessment, particularly in those who are unable to speak [12]. Comorbidities and polypharmacy must be considered and pain management in those with cognitive decline is challenging because of communication difficulties. Good collaboration among the orthogeriatric team is essential for achieving good pain management, particularly so that mobilisation can take place soon after surgery.

Acute pain should be continuously assessed at the time of presentation and then regularly throughout the care pathway so that effective pain management can be implemented. Every nurse should undertake frequent, accurate pain assessment and administer prescribed analgesia, observing its impact and any side effects and reporting these to the MDT. Administration of nerve blocks preoperatively for patients with hip fracture is becoming increasingly common as they minimise the need for opiates, which have multiple risk factors in older frail patients and have been shown to have a significant positive effect on the pain experience [13]. Advanced and specialist nurses increasingly have a role in the administration of nerve blocks both in the ED and in-patient units.

Frequent pain assessment is the foundation for effective pain management, including using an evidence-based tool to conduct an admission interview and a screen of health records to detect pre-existing painful conditions. An initial assessment usually includes location of pain(s), pain descriptors/characteristics of both new acute and existing persistent pain, pain intensity rating at rest and during activity and pain management history (current and past and both pharmacological and non-pharmacological strategies, their relative effectiveness, and any adverse effects experienced by the patient). Common instruments used for pain assessment are the verbal rating scale (VRS) and the visual analogue scale (VAS) for patients with cognitive decline. Older people are often reluctant to acknowledge and report pain.

Therefore, nurses should be alert to signs of the possibility of pain in older people and observe for behavioral and autonomic signs of pain.

Pain should be assessed:

- Immediately upon presentation
- Within 30 min of administering initial analgesia
- Hourly until settled on the ward
- Regularly as part of routine nursing observations throughout admission.

Immediate analgesia should be offered to all patients presenting with suspected hip fracture, including those with cognitive impairment. The choice and dose of analgesia should be age-appropriate, with close monitoring for associated side effects. Analgesia should be sufficient to allow movements necessary for investigations (indicated by ability to tolerate passive external rotation of the leg) and for nursing care and rehabilitation. Paracetamol can be offered every 6 h unless contraindicated with additional opioids if paracetamol alone does not provide sufficient pain relief, using caution if considering using nonsteroidal anti-inflammatory drugs which are often contraindicated in older people. Non-pharmacological therapies are also an integral part of the treatment plan and a variety of options have been shown to be effective individually or in combination with appropriate medications [1]. Selecting strategies that the patient believes in will enhance the effectiveness. Recommended therapies include, but are not limited to:

- Applying ice packs to the hip for 15 min at a time
- Warm blankets and gentle massage
- Cognitive-behavioral strategies: breathing exercises, relaxation therapy, humor, music therapy and socialization/distraction
- Reposition regularly with supportive pillows
- Use an interdisciplinary approach: occupational therapists may provide custom seating, splints or adaptive devices; physiotherapists will assist in individual mobility, exercise and strengthening programs
- Physical activity to improve range of motion, mobility and strength.

Multimodal analgesia can be used to maximise the positive effect of the selected medications while at the same time limiting the associated adverse effects [14]. Older people are more susceptible to adverse medication reactions. However, analgesics can be used safely and effectively when age-related differences in absorption and distributions of these medications, as well as individual risk factors, are considered [12].

Opioid analgesia is a key component in managing hip fracture pain, but there remains wide variability in individual need; opioid requirements decrease with ageing and side effects can impede mobility, impair cognition and interfere with recovery. Other medications such as sedatives, antiemetics and neuroleptics may increase opioid sedation and adverse effects need to be considered when dosing and titrating opioids. It is essential to anticipate and monitor common side effects such as sedation, constipation, nausea and vomiting and instigate preventive treatment as appropriate [15]. Older people have increased risk of respiratory depression with opioids, so regularly monitoring sedation levels is recommended.

Turning the patient with a hip fracture onto the affected side should be avoided until it has been surgically fixed; gently "tipping" the patient may be unavoidable when performing care and checking the skin on the patient's back. Pillows should be used between the thighs and knees to help to manage pain and adduction or rotation of the affected leg should be avoided. Changing the patient's position should always be performed by two experienced nurses using good manual handling practice.

5.6 Postoperative Care

Mobilising the patient soon after surgery has proven to be beneficial in prevention of the complications of mobility and in assisting recovery (Chap. 6). Following surgery, it should be standard practice to sit the patient out of bed and begin to stand them on the day after surgery, providing this is not medically contraindicated. Progress thereafter varies considerably depending on the individual patient and the type of fracture or surgery. Patients with extracapsular fractures tend to take longer than those with intracapsular fractures [9]. Initially, patients may be afraid of weight bearing on the operated leg and should be motivated by the care team, bearing in mind the need for effective pain management.

5.6.1 Pain

Most patients have constant pain in the days following surgery which worsens when they move, so they want to lie still to avoid pain, increasing the risk of immobility. The same principles of pain assessment and pain management discussed earlier apply in the postoperative period. If pain is poorly controlled, mobilisation will be delayed, increasing the risk of the complications of prolonged immobility and leading to increased dependency and associated rise in the risk of delirium [16]. The highly variable nature of pain and an individual's response to it make accurate assessment a central aspect of nursing care to facilitate individualised pain management and monitoring. Many studies have shown that cognitively impaired and acutely confused patients receive less analgesia than their unimpaired counterparts. To help staff understand the individual needs of a person with dementia, the use of an assessment tool to such as the "this is me" tool (Alzheimer's Society (UK) https://www.alzheimers.org.uk/) encourages relatives and carers to share individual information, characteristics and behaviour that enable staff to better understand pain experience and needs. Pain assessment, evaluation, reassessment and appropriate administration of analgesia should be central to routine care.

5.7 Fundamental Nursing Care

Maintaining mobility, energy and participation in self-care during an older person's hospital stay can maintain their independence, reduce the likelihood of falls and fall-related injuries and minimise loss of confidence due to fear of falling (Chap. 3). The underlying principle of quality of care is empathy, a complex multidimensional aspect of the therapeutic relationship involving the ability to understand the needs, meanings, fears, priorities and perspectives of patients [17]. Interaction between the caregiver and a patient with cognitive decline can be a source of stress, particularly if the cognitive impairment (or dementia) sufferer resists the efforts of the caregiver (Chap. 9). Attending to comfort and hygiene is fundamental and includes, for example, acknowledging that patients often feel extreme hunger and thirst and a dry mouth, so effective and frequent mouth care is essential. Many other aspects of fundamental nursing care during the perioperative period are covered in other chapters including:

Acute delirium—the nursing team is most likely to recognise the signs of delirium (Chap. 9).

Pressure injury prevention—pressure injuries are serious complications of immobility, hospitalisation and surgery and can affect up to one third of hip fracture patients [9] (Chap. 7).

Hydration, nutrition, and constipation—fluid management in older people can be difficult as they may self-regulate fluid intake to control incontinence or urinary frequency and to manage difficulties in accessing toilet facilities. Close monitoring of fluid balance is an essential aspect of nursing care to prevent or identify renal injury and patients' acceptance of fluids and nutritional supplement drinks is often poor. Nutrition is linked to all recovery outcomes and is the responsibility of the whole team, but the nursing team is central to adequate dietary intake because of their 24-h presence (Chap. 8).

Constipation—this can be acute or chronic and is a significant and common complication for patients following fracture and during periods of ill health and immobility. Prevention should be considered early in the care pathway; this should involve:

- Regular assessment of bowel function including frequency and consistency of defecation
- Providing and encouraging a fibre-rich but palatable diet
- Careful but early use of prescribed aperients.

Nurses should also educate patients about how to diminish aperients after discharge according to their changed mobility, regained privacy and, eventually, regained appetite.

Healthcare-associated infection—prevention, recognition and management are the responsibility of the whole medical team but are central to 24-h nursing care that often includes coordination of care provided by other team members. Nurses in leadership roles can be instrumental in ensuring adherence of staff to infection prevention guidelines. Prevention of pulmonary infections, urinary tract infections and thromboembolism is also important in perioperative care.

Secondary fracture prevention—an important aspect of preparing the patient for discharge is considering the secondary prevention of the fracture. This is considered in detail in Chaps. 1 and 3 and should be a focus during the entire of the patient's stay in hospital. This includes referral for diagnosis and treatment of osteoporosis and assessment and prevention of falls risk.

5.8 Preparation for Discharge

Discharge planning should be a coordinated effort between the patient, the patient's family, the multidisciplinary team and staff in the destination setting, if the patient is to be discharged to another care facility (Chap. 10). This process should begin as soon as possible following admission. Education of the patient and family or other carers is an important aspect of preparing for discharge. This can be a challenge for healthcare providers because of decreasing lengths of stay and the need to deliver increasingly complex information, so providing patients with alternative ways of receiving information is valuable. The responsibility for the patient's care after discharge from the hospital is often delegated to the patient and their family along with the general practitioner and, sometimes, community care staff. The patient and their caregivers must be able to understand the discharge instructions so that they can recall aftercare instructions and recognise that the information they require for their post-discharge care can be found in their instructions. Providing patients with an information booklet or automated pictographic illustration of discharge instructions have been proven valuable [18–20]. There are several reasons for supporting oral information or education: the older person's visual clarity and auditory acuity decreases, making it difficult for them to receive information and poor lighting, noise levels and room temperatures can inhibit the learning process. Managing multiple messages can be difficult for older people; their personal perception of the severity of their injury and surgery can be significant and pain will limit their ability to receive and understand information. Anticipation, anxiety and fear all contribute to diminished reception of knowledge and fear and preconceived notion of the consequences of acquiring a hip fracture have also been reported to block patients' ability to receive information [6]. These factors need to be taken into consideration when preparing the patient for discharge.

5.9 Summary of Key Points

- The care of the orthogeriatric patient following hip fracture and subsequent surgery presents significant challenges for the healthcare team
- Effective evidence-based nursing care is one of the crucial factors that impact on patient outcomes following hip fracture

- Nurses caring for patients in the perioperative period need to understand different types of hip fracture and their management so that they can deliver evidence-based acute and perioperative care to patientss with hip fracture based on each person's specific needs
- Much of the pre-, peri-, and postoperative care of the patient in need of hip fracture surgery is aimed at maintaining safety and preventing and recognising the complications of the fracture and surgery
- Many aspects of this care are discussed in other chapters within this book as well as summarised here
- Even once the patient has recovered from surgery, there remains the need to comprehensively prepare them for discharge.

5.10 Suggested Further Study

Read the following two journal papers on patients' experiences of acquiring a hip fracture:

- Gesar B et al. (2017). Hip fracture; an interruption that has consequences four months later. A qualitative study. Int J Orthop Trauma Nurs, 26, 43–48. doi:https://doi.org/10.1016/j.ijotn.2017.04.002
- Jensen CM et al. (2017). "If only had I known": a qualitative study investigating a treatment of patients with a hip fracture with short time stay in hospital. Int J Qual Stud Health Well-being, *12*(1):1307061 doi:https://doi.org/10.1080/17482631.2017.1307061

Then write a reflection about what you think is important for patients in their perioperative care.

Talk with your colleagues about what you have learned and the ways you could use this to address the problems identified.

Talk with patients and relatives and other health professionals about topics concerning the patient pathway such as preoperative care and pain management. Reflect on what you learn from these discussions and make suggestions about how practice might be developed to improve satisfaction by involvement of patients and relatives in care.

Further Suggested Reading About Visual and Hearing Impairment

- Berry P, et al. (2004) Vision and hearing loss in older adults: "double trouble", Care Management Journal 5(1):35–40.
- Heine C & Browning CJ (2002) Communication and psychosocial consequences of sensory loss in older adults: overview and rehabilitation directions, Disability and Rehabilitation 24(15):763–773
- Vision Australia (2012) Working with people with vision loss. Vision Australia, Sydney.
- Saxon SV et al. (2009) Physical change and aging: a guide for helping professions, Springer: New York

Further Suggested Reading About Pain Management

- Schug A et al. (2015) Australian and New Zealand College of Anaesthetists and Faculty of Pain Medicine, Acute Pain management: scientific evidence, 4th edn http://fpm.anzca.edu.au/documents/apmse4_2015_final
- British Pain Society and British Geriatric Society (2007) Guidance on: The assessment of pain in older people http://www.bgs.org.uk/Publications/PublicationDownloads/Sep2007PainAssessment.pdf

5.11 How to Self-Assess Learning

To identify learning achieved and the need for further study, the following strategies may be helpful:

- Examine local documentation of nursing care regarding hip fracture care and other outcomes and use this to assess your own knowledge and performance. Fundamentally, nursing is a team effort, so consider this from your own individual perspective as well as that of the team.
- Seek advice and mentorship from other expert clinicians regarding the issues raised in this chapter, e.g. pain specialists, anesthetists, geriatricians and physiotherapists. Have "learning conversations" with specialists and other members of the team to keep up to date on new evidence and disseminate it to colleagues. These conversations can include any recent new practices, guidance, knowledge or evidence.
- Review indicators of good practice (e.g. complication incidence, length of stay) and regularly assess patient and carer views and satisfaction; satisfaction has been recognised as an independent indicator of nursing care quality.
- Peer review by colleagues can be used to assess individual progress and practice but should not be too formal. There should be open discussion within the team. Weekly case conferences can identify nurse-focused issues and enable the exchange of expertise.
- Collaborate with health professionals from other departments covering the patient pathway to undertake case evaluation.

References

1. Maher AB (2012) Acute nursing care of the older adult with fragility hip fracture: an international perspective (Part 1). Int J Orthop Trauma Nurs 16(4):177–194
2. Maher AB et al (2013) Acute nursing care of the older adult with fragility hip fracture: an international perspective (Part 2). Int J Orthop Trauma Nurs 17(1):4–18
3. Handoll HH, Parker MJ (2008) Conservative versus operative treatment for hip fractures in adults. Cochrane Database Syst Rev 3:CD000337
4. Palm H (2017) Hip fracture: the choice of surgery. In: Falaschi P, Marsh D (eds) Orthogeriatrics. Springer, Basel, pp 81–96
5. Gesar B et al (2017) Hip fracture; an interruption that has consequences four months later. A qualitative study. Int J Orthop Trauma Nurs 26:43–48

6. Jensen CM et al (2017) "If only had I known": a qualitative study investigating a treatment of patients with a hip fracture with short time stay in hospital. Int J Qual Stud Health Well-being 12(1):1307061
7. Weissenberger-Leduc M, Zmaritz M (2013) Nursing care for the elderly with hip fracture in an acute care hospital. Wien Med Wochenschr 163(19–20):468–475
8. Curtis E et al (2017) The impact of fragility fracture and approaches to osteoporosis risk assessment worldwide. Bone 104:29–38
9. BOA (British Orthopaedic Association) (2007) The care of patients with fragility facture. BOA, London
10. Zidén L et al (2010) The break remains—elderly people's experiences of a hip fracture 1 year after discharge. Disabil Rehabil 32(2):103–113
11. Ziden L et al (2008) A life-breaking event: early experiences of the consequences of a hip fracture for elderly people. Clin Rehabil 22(9):801–811
12. American Geriatrics Society (2009) American Geriatrics Society panel on persistent pain in older persons. Pharmacological management of persistent pain in older persons. J Am Geriatr Soc 57: 1331–1346
13. Obideyi A et al (2008) Nurse administered fascia iliaca compartment block for pre-operative pain relief in adult fractured neck of femur. Acute Pain 10(3):145–149
14. Kehlet H, Dahl JB (2003) Anaesthesia, surgery, and challenges in postoperative recovery. Lancet 362(9399):1921–1928
15. Registered Nurses' Association of Ontario. Assessment and management of pain. Nursing best practice guideline. 3rd edn, 2013. http://rnao.ca/sites/rnao-ca/files/AssessAndManagementOfPain2014.pdf
16. Bjorkelund KB et al (2010) Reducing delirium in elderly patients with hip fracture: a multifactorial intervention study. Acta Anaesthesiol Scan 54:678–688
17. Mercer SW, Reynolds WJ (2002) Empathy and quality of care. Br J Gen Pract 52(Suppl):S9–S12
18. Choi J (2013) Improving discharge education using pictographs. Rehabil Nurs 38(5):240–246
19. Hill B et al (2016) Automated pictographic illustration of discharge instructions with glyph: impact on recall and satisfaction. J Am Med Inform Assoc 23(6):1136–1142
20. Murphy S et al (2011) An intervention study exploring the effects of providing older adult hip fracture patients with an information booklet in the early postoperative period. J Clin Nurs 20(23–24):3404–3413

6 Mobility, Remobilisation, Exercise and Prevention of the Complications of Stasis

Panagiota Copanitsanou

The positive effects of physical activity on physical and mental health are well known and include weight control, improved balance, flexibility, strength, anxiety reduction and protection from ill health, as well as contributing to independent living and preventing falls. Being mobile and able to self-care and fear of falling are important to patients. A central goal of nursing care following fragility fracture is to maximise mobility. Individual patient goals are determined by their pre-fracture mobility and functional status. Recovery is often compromised for those with limited pre-fracture activity and cognitive impairment, low functional levels postoperatively, older age, polypharmacy, comorbidities, depression, poor nutritional status, lack of social support and not living independently. Many patients never recover their previous level of function after a fragility fracture and there is significant risk of institutionalisation, new fractures, disability and loss of independence.

Patients should undergo multidisciplinary assessment to identify factors known to be associated with risk for poor functional recovery so that appropriate multidisciplinary interventions can be implemented. The aim of this chapter is to highlight the risks of immobility and the benefits of remobilisation and exercise to enable clinicians to effectively manage the multiple and interconnected individual factors of each patient to maximise their function.

P. Copanitsanou
Department of Orthopaedic and Traumatology, General Hospital of Piraeus "Tzaneio", Piraeus, Greece

National and Kapodistrian University of Athens, Athens, Greece
e-mail: gcopanitsan@nurs.uoa.gr

K. Hertz, J. Santy-Tomlinson (eds.), *Fragility Fracture Nursing*, Perspectives in Nursing Management and Care for Older Adults, https://doi.org/10.1007/978-3-319-76681-2_6

6.1 Learning Outcomes

At the end of the chapter, and following further study, the nurse will be able to:

- Identify the risks of immobilisation and benefits of remobilisation and exercise
- Highlight the importance of mobilisation and exercise in the prevention of complications and effective recovery
- Recognise the factors that affect mobility
- Define which factors must be considered when assessing patients' mobility and capacity for remobilisation and exercise
- Describe the most effective approach for pain assessment and management
- Define the relationship between immobility and stasis and complications following hip fracture
- Outline the evidence-based measures for the prevention of venous thromboembolism, urinary tract infection, constipation and pneumonia
- Implement appropriate exercises and mobilisation strategies and document care
- Confidently support older people with fragility fractures in their difficult journey to recovery.

6.2 Mobility and Remobilisation

Mobilisation is essential for health-related quality of life and independence. For older people following hip fracture, early mobilisation is especially important because it is linked to mortality [1] and functional recovery [2] as well as risk of functional decline due to the injury, perioperative immobilisation, muscle weakness, fatigue and postoperative complications.

Pain limits remobilisation and is associated with delirium, depression, sleep disturbances and poor mobility. Muscle strength deficit in the fractured limb is associated with even greater pain and it is unethical to expect patients to comply with rehabilitation exercises without managing pain effectively. Good pain management helps avoid delays in rehabilitation, postoperative complications, delayed discharge and unsafe mobility.

Patients also suffer from loss of confidence, fear of falling and are at risk of further fractures and other complications. Older women have been found to prefer being dead than experience loss of independence [3], demonstrating the psychological impact. Those who are not remobilised early may feel demoralised, so it is important that they have realistic expectations to avoid disappointment. Management of the fear of falling is also central, along with the need to educate patients and carers about fall prevention and the importance of exercise.

There are numerous factors that affect ability to remobilise. The progressive loss of muscle mass with ageing is associated with decreasing reserves and sarcopenia (Chap. 2) as well as immobility. For every day spent in bed, 2.5 days are needed to regain the strength to walk [4]. Frailty leads to poor outcomes and affects capacity for mobilisation and exercise. Other conditions to consider include depression, cognitive impairment and delirium (Chap. 9), which are also associated with poorer mobility outcomes and limit participation in exercise. The main factors that impact on ability to remobilise are summarised in Box 6.1.

It is essential to consider the impact of these multiple factors on exercise and mobility and take an individualised, holistic approach. Patients who were mobile before the fracture should be mobilised regardless of their cognitive status and the focus should be on gait quality, walking endurance, activities of daily living and safety [5].

Box 6.1: Factors Affecting Ability to Mobilise After Fragility Fracture

- Pain
- Loss of confidence, fear of falling, fear of refracturing the bone, fear of other local/ surgical complications
- Osteoporosis
- Comorbidities, multimorbidity
- Polypharmacy
- Nutritional status
- Progressive muscle loss, sarcopenia
- Frailty
- Cognitive impairment, depression, delirium

6.3 Exercise

Mobilisation strategy, type of weight bearing, timing and progress of exercise depend on the type of fracture and surgery and there are contradictions about evidence-based pathways for management after different fractures and procedures; e.g. after hemiarthroplasty, mobilisation may start earlier, while following extracapsular fracture, it may be delayed. Surgeons usually decide when to allow restricted or full weight bearing [6], with a mean time for an order for ambulation of 2 days, as some hesitate because of concerns about mechanical failure [7]. However, delay in weight bearing has been connected to poor function [8]. With current implants and surgical techniques, most patients can be allowed to weight bear and movements (e.g. crossing the legs past the midline of the body, avoiding bending or overreaching) should not be restricted. Familiarity with basic exercises (i.e. foot and ankle, static quadricep/gluteal/abdominal, knee extension/flexion, hip abduction) as well as functional exercises is essential. However, walking may be compromised by practical obstacles such as wound drains, intravenous infusion devices and the surgical wound.

Nurses should encourage patients to sit in a chair for meals as soon as possible and encourage them to be independent in self-care and hygiene. All staff should be involved in encouraging independence in toileting and transfers and in making daily assessments of patients' progress so that they can determine individual needs and prevent delays in transfers and discharge.

Effective pain management is central in enabling patients to exercise, sleep well and promote recovery. A baseline pain assessment (pain history, previous use of pain medications) should be performed, and mobilisation and pain management should be coordinated (i.e. correct timing of medication administration in relation to exercise sessions). Patients' self-report is the gold standard for assessing pain. Assessment should be conducted using numerical, verbal, facial, or visual analogue scales. Adjustments in medication dose may be needed based on individual responses, as some patients may become sedated, while others may need higher doses. Pain management interventions should not only be pharmacological but also include non-pharmacological options such as transcutaneous electrical nerve stimulation, distraction, muscle relaxation, acupressure, heat/ice and relaxation techniques. Multiple strategies should be used in combination. A self-reported reduction of pain by 20–30% is considered effective [9].

Patients do not always receive adequate pain management, especially those with dementia and/or delirium who have more difficulty reporting pain [10], and behavioural (e.g. moans, sighs, restlessness, agitation, rapid blinking, facial expressions) or physiological (e.g. tachycardia, high blood pressure) signs are rarely considered. Effective pain assessment requires familiarity with the patient and information from carers [11]. Pain may not only be acute (up to 30 days postfracture/surgery) but may also be chronic [9]. Although some discomfort is expected during the first few months, patients must be able to differentiate between discomfort and pain [4]. Nurses should inform patients about when increased pain indicates a problem and about the avoidance of exercise when strain on the surgical area is experienced.

To minimise the risk for falling (Chap. 3) and for remobilisation to be safe, patients should be actively involved in their own care. Assistance should be provided as needed for them to remain as functional and active as possible. Even if they cannot perform exercises alone, they must not remain immobilised but should undertake simple exercises in bed or while sitting in a chair. Nurses need to know how to help patients to mobilise safely as in-hospital falls are a nursing care quality indicator.

Patient education should include the type of pain medications and time intervals for administration, the importance of receiving medications before the pain becomes intense, coordination between the administration of pain medication and exercise and the interactions of medications. Patients should be reminded that exercise helps to reduce pain and that pain improves more quickly if they stay active and achieve a balance between activity and rest [4].

6.4 The Complications of Stasis

Nearly half of patients with a hip fracture develop at least one complication [12]. Surgical management enables earlier mobilisation and prevents complications of prolonged immobilisation (e.g., urinary tract infections, pressure ulcers, respiratory/cardiac/renal/gastrointestinal complications, venous thromboembolism).

6.4.1 Venous Thromboembolism

Deep vein thrombosis (DVT) following hip fracture has a frequency of 1–24%, depending on the screening method used, while the frequency of fatal pulmonary embolism ranges between 0.5 and -7.5% [10]. Patients with fragility fracture are susceptible to venous thromboembolism (VTE) due to ageing, the fracture itself, immobilisation, hospitalisation and surgery. Other risk factors include history of previous thromboembolism, malignancy, congestive heart failure, obesity and vascular disease.

6.4.2 Pulmonary and Urinary Tract Infection

Hospital-acquired infections cause significant morbidity and must be prevented. Postoperatively, pulmonary complications are among the most frequent and their occurrence can increase from 6.3% preoperatively to 10.7% postoperatively [13]. Complications such as atelectasis and pneumonia contribute to increased length of hospital stay and mortality [14]. The risk factors for the development of a pulmonary infection include chronic respiratory disease, male gender, use of steroids, number of comorbidities and older age [15].

The frequency of urinary tract infections (UTI) has been reported to be as low as 2% [13] and as high as 52% [16]. UTI is associated with increased length of hospital stay and poor functional outcomes and is usually caused by the use of indwelling catheters. Urinary catheters also cause restriction of mobility, pain, delirium and increased mortality [17].

Indwelling urinary catheters are often inserted on admission or are used postoperatively to accommodate the patients' limited independence. However, the reason for inserting an indwelling catheter is often unclear [18] and should be specifically recorded, e.g. urinary retention unrelieved by intermittent catheterisation, skin problems in the perineal area/sacrum area, for close monitoring of cardiac or renal function or as a comfort measure in end of life care [17]. Patients with indwelling catheters are more likely to have positive urine cultures compared to following intermittent catheterisation [18] and the risk of UTI increases an estimated 5–10% for every 48 h of indwelling urinary catheter placement [19]. Those most at risk are older patients, women [20], those with dehydration and/or poor nutrition postoperatively [21] and those with diabetes or malignancy [13].

6.4.3 Constipation

Constipation often occurs postoperatively because of analgesics, limited activity and lack of privacy but is a commonly overlooked aspect of care; 69% of patients with fragility fractures develop constipation during the first postoperative days and 62% at 30 days after surgery. In 22.7% of patients, a normal defecation pattern may not be re-established even within 30 days [22]. Risk factors include dehydration, immobility, decreased dietary fibre, changes to normal dietary routines and opioid analgesics (even in low doses). Opioid-induced constipation may cause patients to refuse pain medications, thus compromising pain relief and remobilisation. Patients may not inform nurses of their constipation symptoms and nurses may not initiate a conversation. The presence of constipation, symptoms, use of laxatives and impact on pain management is often not fully appreciated by healthcare professionals.

6.5 Assessment of Mobility and Remobilisation Potential

Mobility status affects patient handling and outcomes, so mobility, remobilisation and exercise ability should be carefully assessed taking into account patients' function, cognitive and psychosocial status. Due to their 24-hour presence and ability to perform continuous assessment of progress, nurses do not need to rely on other healthcare professionals to determine patients' mobility. The criteria for assessing mobility are subjective because quantifiable terms for mobility are rarely used. A summary of factors to consider when assessing mobility is provided in Box 6.2.

Assessing mobility using tests for physical function (e.g. range of motion) is limited, as tests may be unreliable between different observers. Likewise, the observation of mobilisation can be intrusive or may only convey "snapshots" of patients' abilities unless observation takes place on several occasions over a period of time. By interviewing patients, information can be gathered about their views regarding their situation, strengths and problems, but even this may be compromised by difficulties in communication and by patients' cognitive impairment as well as their desire to appear better than they are [23].

Several tools have been developed for assessment of mobility and remobilisation ability. Options include the New Mobility Score, the Quick 5 Bedside Guide tool, the Hand Grip measurement, the Berg Balance Scale, the de Morton Mobility Index, the Modified Elderly Mobility Scale, the Timed Up and Go Test, the Banner Mobility Assessment Tool, the Tinetti Assessment Tool, the Barthel Index, the Egress Test, the Functional Independence Measure, the Functional Assessment Measure, the Performance-Oriented Mobility Assessment and the Elderly Mobility Scale. Although these tools are used in hospitals, they may be inappropriate or of limited value for nurses in acute-care settings. There is a need to understand how they should be used and their validity, reliability and practicability, as well as any copyright restrictions. The information gathered can help to inform history taking and can be used to compare and document progress throughout rehabilitation [23].

The assessment of mobility potential has not only to do with mobility itself but includes individual goals, safety and use of appropriate walking aids. Safety is an important parameter and nurses need to know how to assess individual risks, how to manage them, how to use appropriate aids, how to safely handle each patient and how to ensure the environment is safe.

Other, more targeted, assessments may include that of the musculoskeletal system (e.g. muscle mass/strength, sarcopenia, presence of arthritis, osteoporosis, neuromusculoskeletal disorders), pre-fracture mobility and lifestyle (e.g. dependent, sedentary, independent), cognitive and psychosocial status, any visual and/or hearing disorders, the presence of significant others, the patient's own beliefs and willingness for mobilisation and their educational needs regarding mobility/remobilisation.

Box 6.2: Assessment of Mobility and Remobilisation Potential

- General physical health status
- Assessment of musculoskeletal system (e.g. muscle mass/strength, sarcopenia, presence of arthritis, osteoporosis, neuro-musculoskeletal disorders)
- Pain
- Lifestyle before the fracture (dependent, sedentary, independent)
- Cognitive status, depression, delirium
- Visual and/or hearing disorders
- Presence of family/significant others
- Patient's beliefs and willingness for remobilisation
- Educational needs regarding mobility/remobilisation

6.6 Evidence-Based Interventions for Mobility and Remobilisation

Rehabilitation should start as soon as possible postoperatively once the patient is medically stable. There is a series of actions that nurses need to perform both as members of the multidisciplinary team (MDT) and independently to promote this (a summary is provided in Box 6.3). Through patient-centred participation and collaboration with the MDT and with the patient participating in the goal-setting, nurses help to set individual and realistic goals and plan interventions that support individual preferences and actively encourage patients in self-care and independence. When a patient is transferred or discharged, nurses should communicate any successful strategies or risks observed during hospitalisation to other healthcare professionals [5].

Nurses play a key role in the patients' psychological and biophysiological preparation for remobilisation and they can provide sustained encouragement. Through therapeutic communication with patients, nurses can ensure they are treated as individuals and that they are supported after their great trauma towards a future of independent life and to believe in the possibility that this is achievable. In acute trauma wards, there is often limited opportunity for physical activity [24], but nurses can encourage patients to remain physically active and participate in self-care so that functional decline is reduced [25].

Patient education, as an independent nursing intervention, can be used to inform patients about the importance of mobilisation and exercise, complication prevention, rehabilitation programme and long-term outcomes. Education helps motivate patients to want to move, as they are often reluctant to comply with rehabilitation. Nurses need to be firm in encouraging them to move, but at the same time, they should make sure they do so without patronising them. The anxieties of patients and their carers should be recognised and addressed. Family members provide a support network that enhances patient recovery through practical help and psychosocial support and can be a valuable source of information about the patient's pre-fracture status and preferences [24]. High-quality care of older patients relies not only on excellent MDT communication but also on close cooperation with patients and families.

Box 6.3: Evidence-Based Interventions for Mobility and Remobilisation

- Encouraging and supporting in remobilisation, self-care and independence
- Use of safety measures/prevention of falls/walking aids
- Education about exercises (both of patients and family/carers)
- Pain management (before remobilisation)
- Adequate rest/sleep
- Adequate nutrition/hydration
- Participation within the multidisciplinary team (patient-centred)
- Communication of any successful strategies or risks observed during hospitalisation to other healthcare professionals after discharge

6.7 Exercise: Assessment

Before the commencement of exercise, there should be an overall assessment of functional level, ability to perform Activities of Daily Living (ADLs) and the assistance needed to accomplish them, sensory ability, cognitive status and capacity to ambulate. This should include an evaluation of gait instability and risk of falls. Older people often view their health in terms of how well they function, not in terms of disease, and it is important to identify strengths as well as need for assistance. Baseline functional status should be documented to facilitate assessment of progress. Assessment should also include information about the type of fracture and surgery (to determine what exercise is feasible or unadvisable) and the needs for walking aids and personal safety measures. For example, the selection of the most appropriate walking stick should be made according to the fracture type as well as hand grip, gait, height and stability.

6.8 Exercise: Evidence-Based Interventions

Mobilising patients early leads to reduced length of hospital stay, improved mobility, improved walking distance and overall improved function [26, 27]. Although patients with good pre-fracture level of mobility without cognitive impairment tend to benefit most from rehabilitation, exercise is beneficial even in the presence of functional limitations and/or cognitive impairment [2, 28]. It is essential to increase muscle strength and range of motion [9], so walking and exercise training aim to minimise impairment [6]. The type, frequency and duration of exercise that is recommended postoperatively (sometimes after x-rays to check the stability of fixation and the surgeon's agreement) for each patient are also important factors. Remobilisation should start with simple exercises, while their intensity gradually progress.

There is some evidence that exercise with higher intensity and duration is related to better outcomes [28], while potential risks of intensive exercise appear to be minimal. Specific types of exercises are beneficial such as progressive resistance training and balance training, which can be safe and effective [29]. However, there is insufficient evidence about the best strategies for enhancing mobility and more research is needed to determine the most appropriate type, duration and intensity of exercise, as well as the value of first-day mobilisation.

There are several ways for nurses to help patients comply with exercise programmes and maximise performance. They can encourage patients to maintain a daily routine with physical activity; they can educate them on the physiological and psychological value of independent functioning, assess and treat their pain, ensure a safe environment, emphasise the importance of nutrition and medications and document all interventions and responses.

6.9 Prevention of Complications of Stasis

Complications may be caused by limited mobility and, in a vicious circle, they can limit mobilisation potential due to pain, distress and restrictions caused by treatment or safety measures. They can also lead to poorer outcomes and mortality.

6.9.1 Assessment

As part of the prevention strategy, patients should be assessed for the presence of signs and symptoms of thromboembolism which can be nonspecific but include pain (especially during dorsiflexion of the foot), tenderness, changes in colour and temperature of the skin, oedema and, in the case of pulmonary embolism; dyspnoea, chest pain, increased respiratory rate and haemoptysis. However, even in the presence of pulmonary embolism, there may be no signs or symptoms, with cardiac arrest being the first manifestation. Medical history and a physical examination should be used to exclude other causes.

Assessment is important in identifying individual risk of pulmonary infections such as being of older age, poor general health, other infections, cardiopulmonary diseases, malnutrition and impaired renal function [14]. Nurses should assess for presence of cough, sputum production, increased respiratory rate, oxygen saturation levels, dyspnoea, elevated temperature, pleuritic pain, rhonchi/wheezes, use of accessory breathing muscles, cyanosis and changes in mental status.

Assessment for UTI should include monitoring for fever, burning during urination/dysuria, urgency and frequency of urination, suprapubic or pelvic pain, haematuria and new onset or worsening of pre-existing confusion/agitation. Urine colour, concentration, odour, reduced volume and cloudiness should also be assessed. The presence of asymptomatic bacteriuria, especially in older people, does not necessitate treatment.

Assessment for constipation should include the number of bowel movements per day/week, abdominal distention and discomfort, abdominal or rectal pain, decreased appetite, nausea, vomiting, bowel obstruction, headache, fatigue, agitation and delirium. Nurses should document usual bowel patterns, severity of constipation and any improvements or progression of constipation [17].

6.9.2 Prevention of Complications

The prevention of complications enables patients to participate actively in rehabilitation. There is evidence in favour of mobilisation to prevent thromboembolism and urinary tract infections.

6.9.2.1 Prevention of Thromboembolism

There is insufficient evidence for a protocol to be developed regarding thromboembolic prophylaxis following hip fracture. Aspirin significantly reduces DVT and pulmonary embolism (PE) compared to placebo, and, although patients treated with aspirin need more blood transfusions, mortality associated with bleeding is similar. Nevertheless, aspirin is inferior to other methods of prophylaxis. The overall balance of risks and benefits is complex in hip fracture patients [30].

It has been shown that the administration of heparin leads to a reduction in the frequency of lower limb thromboembolism, but not PE, and there seems to be no difference in efficacy between fractionated or unfractionated heparins; low molecular weight heparins have improved bioavailability, have fewer side effects and are easy to use. Treatment usually takes place for 28–35 days. Both low molecular weight heparins and unfractionated heparin should start on admission unless contraindicated, stoped 12 h preoperatively and restarted 6–12 h postoperatively [30]. Guidelines state that chemoprophylaxis with fondaparinux should continue for 4 weeks after surgery. Fondaparinux seems to be more efficient than low molecular weight heparins in preventing thromboembolism without significant differences in mortality or bleeding. However, it is not recommended for preoperative use in patients with hip fractures; if it is used preoperatively, it should be stopped 24 h before surgery and restarted 6 h postoperatively [30].

Mechanical prophylaxis is also recommended for prevention of thromboembolism, should start on admission and should be continued until mobility has been restored. Intermittent pneumatic compression (foot impulse devices) can reduce the risk of VTE. Anti-embolism stockings are effective but are difficult, and sometimes painful, to put on and can cause skin injury in people with fragile skin or vascular insufficiency, or if the stockings are ill-fitting [11]. Nurses should be trained in how to use mechanical prophylaxis and encourage patients to comply.

Other recommended measures to reduce the risk of VTE include the avoidance of dehydration, early surgery, avoidance of prolonged surgery, avoidance of over transfusion and early mobilisation [31]. Early mobilisation is simple and particularly effective in lowering the risk of thrombosis, as it increases blood flow, prevents the formation of clots and has an impact on physiological and psychological health with no bleeding complications. Simple exercises, such as walking, repositioning, calf pump exercises and deep breathing help prevent venous stasis [4] and both active and passive leg exercises should be performed to increase blood flow.

6.9.2.2 Prevention of Pulmonary Infections

Early remobilisation is central in the prevention of pneumonia [6, 32]. Techniques such as lung expansion manoeuvres (e.g. deep breathing, spirometry) can also reduce the risk of pulmonary complications [14]. Treatment, in addition to antibiotic therapy, includes hydration, a high-calorie/high-protein diet, administration of antipyretics and bronchodilators, rest, oxygen therapy in the case of hypoxemia, monitoring of respiratory status and general health, encouragement of coughing and deep breathing. Patients should be positioned in semi-Fowler position to facilitate breathing, while repositioning helps in loosening lung secretions.

6.9.2.3 Prevention of Urinary Tract Infection (UTI)

UTIs are preventable and early identification of infection leads to prompt treatment and improved outcomes. Early mobilisation is central in prevention and enables patients to maintain self-care and independence while facilitating early removal of catheters. The most important interventions are those of prevention and these are presented in Box 6.4. On suspicion of urinary infection a urine sample should be sent for culture and microbiological analysis followed by appropriate antibiotic therapy. Any indwelling urinary catheter should be removed or replaced before antibiotic administration. Whenever possible, catheters should be avoided or, at least, maintained only for the first 24–48 h postoperatively. If a catheter is retained for more than 24 h, the reason should be documented and removal should take place as soon as possible, followed by monitoring the patient for retention/incontinence.

6.9.2.4 Prevention of Constipation

The prevention and treatment of constipation involves documentation of stool type (e.g. using the Bristol Stool Scale) and bowel function (e.g. Bowel Function Index), maintaining good nutrition and hydration status, minimising anxiety and maintaining patients' privacy. The overuse of laxatives is a problem which should not be underestimated. The effectiveness of different laxatives does not differ significantly, but the treatment is usually not adjusted satisfactorily to individual needs [33]. Laxatives may not be necessary for patients who are well hydrated and follow a diet rich in fibre (these patients are also more likely to be well nourished) [34]. Prevention and treatment of constipation can also be assisted by good access to toilet facilities, minimising fasting periods and encouraging exercise/mobility. A regular toileting regime (e.g. every 2 h) that encourages ambulation and discourages the use of bedpans and an aim for a bowel movement by the second postoperative day (then every 48 h) can also assist in prevention [35], but individual patients will differ in what is normal for them.

Box 6.4: Summary of Evidence-Based Interventions for the Prevention/ Management of the Complications of Stasis

Deep vein thrombosis

- Risk factors: older age, previous thromboembolism, malignancy, congestive heart failure, obesity, deep venous system disease, surgery, long immobilisation, dehydration
- Assessment: pain, tenderness, changes in skin colour/temperature, oedema (pulmonary embolism: dyspnoea, chest pain, increased respiratory rate, coughing up blood)
- Heparin treatment (low molecular weight/unfractionated)
- Fondaparinux
- Mechanical prophylaxis (intermittent pneumatic compression/foot impulse devices, anti-embolism stockings)
- Avoidance of dehydration
- Early surgery, avoidance of prolonged surgery
- Avoidance of over transfusion
- Early mobilisation

Pulmonary and urinary infections

- Risk factors: older age, poor general health, other infections, cardiopulmonary disease, low albumin, impaired renal function)
- Assessment: cough, sputum production, breaths per minute, type of breathing, saturation levels, dyspnoea, chills, elevated temperature, pleuritic pain, rhonchi/wheezes, use of accessory breathing muscles, cyanosis, mental status
- Techniques such as lung expansion exercises (e.g. deep breathing, spirometry)
- Early ambulation postoperatively
- Hydration, high-calorie/high-protein diet, administration of antipyretics and bronchodilators, rest, oxygen therapy, monitoring, encouragement of coughing/deep breathing
- Semi-Fowler position to facilitate breathing
- Repositioning

Urinary tract infections

- Risk factors: indwelling catheters, older patients, women, dehydration, poor nutrition, diabetes, malignancy
- Assessment: fever, burning during urination/dysuria, urgency and frequency of urination, suprapubic/pelvic pain, haematuria, onset/worsening

of pre-existing confusion/agitation, urine characteristics (colour, concentration, odour, volume, cloudiness)
- Catheters need not to be put at admission as standard procedure-intermittent catheterisation instead of indwelling catheters
- Analgesic medications administered in the presence of pain
- Good hydration
- Recording of input and output
- Removal of catheters as early as possible postoperatively (after removal, monitoring for retention/incontinence)
- Early identification of infection, prompt treatment
- Preserving functional ability to increase independence and self-care
- Sterile technique for insertion and care:
  - Use of lubricant from a single-use container
  - Insertion of the smallest lumen catheter possible and instilling 5 mL in the balloon
  - Ensuring that catheter is properly secured (in the abdomen/thigh) to minimise trauma
  - Use of closed drainage system
  - Sampling port
  - Positioning of the drainage system below the level of bladder
  - Use of separate clean containers to empty each patient's drainage bag (the bag should not be allowed to fill more than 75%)
  - Encourage/perform routine daily personal hygiene
  - Routine catheter care

Constipation

- Risk factors: pain medications, eating habits, limited activity, lack of privacy
- Assessment: number of bowel movements per week, abdominal distention/discomfort, abdominal/rectal pain, decreased appetite, nausea, vomiting, bowel obstruction, headache, fatigue, agitation, delirium
- Good nutritional and hydration status (minimum of 1500 mL of oral fluid daily unless contraindicated)—diet rich in fibre
- Minimisation of extended fasting periods
- Minimisation of anxiety
- Maintaining privacy
- Good accessibility to toilet facilities
- Encouraging exercise and mobility [regular toileting regime (every 2 h) that encourages ambulation and discourages the use of bedpans]
- Administration of laxatives

6.10 Summary of Key Points

- Immobility is associated with poor health outcomes and mobilisation and exercise should be encouraged and individualised
- Individual patient goals are determined by pre-fracture mobility/functional status
- Remobilisation is limited by pain, fear and other factors associated with the fall and fracture so mobilisation and pain management should be coordinated
- Rehabilitation should begin as early as possible
- Assessment includes physical function, family/carer involvement, patient beliefs and motivation, education needs and progress towards goals
- Nurses can reduce the risk of falls, assist with mobilisation, ensure walking aids are used and psychologically support patients and carers, but there is insufficient evidence to establish the best strategies for mobility
- Vigilant assessment, prompt interventions and mobilisation prevent the development of complications
- Mechanical prophylaxis along with chemoprophylaxis is recommended for prevention of thromboembolism
- There are simple evidence-based interventions for the prevention of urinary tract infections and constipation.

6.11 Suggested Further Study

- Read the following journal papers about the experience of hip fracture:
  - Griffiths F et al. (2015) Evaluating recovery following hip fracture: a qualitative interview study of what is important to patients. BMJ Open 5(1):e005406.
  - Sims-Gould J, et al. (2017) Patient Perspectives on Engagement in Recovery after Hip Fracture: A Qualitative Study. J Aging Res. Article ID 2171865 https://doi.org/10.1155/2017/2171865

Then write a reflection about what you have learned that relates to mobility and the way in which you and your team practice in relation to helping patients to remobilise. Talk with your colleagues about what you have found and the ways you could use to address possible problems.

- Talk with patients, carers and other staff about the things they feel prevent active remobilisation following surgery. Reflect on what these conversations suggest about how practice might be developed to improve mobility outcomes by involving patients.

6.12 Self-Assessment

To identify learning achieved and the need for further study, the following strategies may be helpful:

- Examine local documentation of nursing care, regarding mobility status and other outcomes and use this to assess knowledge and performance. There is controversy regarding whether the assessment should be of individual nurses or of the nursing team, as, fundamentally, nursing is a team job.
- Seek advice and mentorship from other expert clinicians.
- Meet with specialists and other members of the team to keep up to date on new evidence and disseminate it to colleagues. The conversation in these meetings can include any recent new practices, guidance, knowledge or evidence.
- Review indicators of good practice (e.g. complications incidence, length of stay) and regularly assess patient and carer views and satisfaction. Patient satisfaction has been recognised as an independent indicator of nursing care quality.
- Peer review by colleagues can be used to assess individual progress and practice but should not be too formal. There should be open discussion within the team. Weekly case conferences can identify nurse-focused issues and enable the exchange of expertise. Expertise is conveyed to the various members of the multidisciplinary team by educational initiatives, and by fostering a culture where all the patients' problems are considered.
- There is a lack of published performance indicators and assessment of practical nursing quality, although certain "never events" have been established by nursing associations.

References

1. Dubljanin Raspopovic E et al (2012) Use of early indicators in rehabilitation process to predict one-year mortality in elderly hip fracture patients. Hip Int 22:661–667
2. Lee D et al (2014) Prognostic factors predicting early recovery of pre-fracture functional mobility in elderly patients with hip fracture. Ann Rehabil Med 38(6):827–835
3. Salkeld G et al (2000) Quality of life related to fear of falling and hip fracture in older women: a time trade off study. BMJ 320(7231):341–346
4. Nurses Improving Care for Healthsystem Elders (NICHE) (2017) NICHE "Need to knows". http://www.nicheprogram.org/need-to-knows/. Accessed 11 July 2017
5. Maher A et al (2012) Acute nursing care of the older adult with fragility hip fracture: an international perspective (part 1). Int J Orthop Trauma Nurs 16:177–194
6. Handoll HH et al (2011) Interventions for improving mobility after hip fracture surgery in adults. Cochrane Database Syst Rev (3):CD001704
7. Kamel HK et al (2003) Time to ambulation after hip fracture surgery: relation to hospitalization outcomes. J Gerontol A Biol Sci Med Sci 58(11):1042–1045

8. Kondo A et al (2010) Determinants of ambulatory ability after hip fracture surgery in Japan and the USA. Nurs Health Sci 12:336–344
9. Abou-Setta AM et al (2011) Comparative effectiveness of pain management interventions for hip fracture: a systematic review. Ann Intern Med 155(4):234–245
10. Egol KA, Strauss EJ (2009) Perioperative considerations in geriatric patients with hip fracture: what is the evidence? J Orthop Trauma 23(6):386–394
11. British Orthopaedic Association (BOA) (2007) The care of patients with fragility fracture. British Orthopaedic Association, London
12. Colón-Emeric CS (2012) Postoperative management of hip fractures: interventions associated with improved outcomes. Bonekey Rep 1:241
13. Copanitsanou P et al (2012) Predictive factors for in-hospital stay and complications after hip fracture. Int J Orthop Trauma Nurs 16:206–213
14. Lo IL et al (2010) Pre-operative pulmonary assessment for patients with hip fracture. Osteoporos Int 21(Suppl 4):S579–S586
15. Roche JJ et al (2005) Effect of comorbidities and postoperative complications on mortality after hip fracture in elderly people: prospective observational cohort study. BMJ 331(7529):1374
16. Halleberg Nyman M et al (2011) A prospective study of nosocomial urinary tract infection in hip fracture patients. J Clin Nurs 20(17–18):2531–2539
17. Maher A et al (2013) Acute nursing care of the older adult with fragility hip fracture: an international perspective (Part 2). Int J Orthop Trauma Nurs 17(1):4–18
18. Johansson I et al (2002) Intermittent versus indwelling catheters for older patients with hip fractures. J Clin Nurs 11(5):651–656
19. Wald H et al (2005) Extended use of indwelling urinary catheters in postoperative hip fracture patients. Med Care 43(10):1009–1017
20. Polites SF et al (2014) Urinary tract infection in elderly trauma patients: review of the Trauma Quality Improvement Program identifies the population at risk. J Trauma Acute Care Surg 77(6):952–959
21. Kamel HK (2005) The frequency and factors linked to a urinary tract infection coding in patients undergoing hip fracture surgery. J Am Med Dir Assoc 6(5):316–320
22. Trads M, Pedersen PU (2015) Constipation and defecation pattern the first 30 days after hip fracture. Int J Nurs Pract 21(5):598–604
23. Jester R (2007) Evaluating rehabilitation services. In: Jester R (ed) Advancing practice in rehabilitation nursing. Wiley-Blackwell, Oxford
24. Riemen AHK, Hutchison JD (2016) The multidisciplinary management of hip fractures in older patients. Orthop Trauma 30(2):117–122
25. Resnick B et al (2015) Optimizing physical activity among older adults post trauma: overcoming system and patient challenges. Int J Orthop Trauma Nurs 19:194–206
26. Healee DJ et al (2011) Older adult's recovery from hip fracture: a literature review. Int J Orthop Trauma Nurs 15:18–28
27. Perme C et al (2014) A tool to assess mobility status in critically ill patients: The Perme Intensive Care Unit Mobility Score. Methodist Debakey Cardiovasc J 10(1):41–49
28. Beaupre LA et al (2013) Maximising functional recovery following hip fracture in frail seniors. Best Pract Res Clin Rheumatol 27(6):771–788
29. Sylliaas H et al (2011) Progressive strength training in older patients after hip fracture: a randomised controlled trial. Age Ageing 40:221–227
30. National Institute for Health and Clinical Excellence (NICE) (2015) Reducing venous thromboembolism risk: orthopaedic surgery. http://pathways.nice.org.uk/pathways/venous-thromboembolism/reducing-venous-thromboembolism-risk-orthopaedic-surgery#content=view-node%3Anodes-hip-fracture
31. Parker M, Johansen A (2006) Hip fracture. BMJ 333(7557):27–30
32. Stolbrink M et al (2014) The early mobility bundle: a simple enhancement of therapy which may reduce incidence of hospital-acquired pneumonia and length of hospital stay. J Hosp Infect 88(1):34–39

33. Fosnes GS et al (2011) Effectiveness of laxatives in elderly—a cross sectional study in nursing homes. BMC Geriatr 11:76
34. Sturtzel B et al (2009) Use of fiber instead of laxative treatment in a geriatric hospital to improve the wellbeing of seniors. J Nutr Health Aging 13(2):136–139
35. Mihaylov S et al (2008) Stepped treatment of older adults on laxatives. The STOOL trial. Health Technol Assess 12(13):iii–iiv, ix-139

Pressure Injury Prevention and Wound Management

7

Ami Hommel and Julie Santy-Tomlinson

The management of wounds and the prevention of pressure injuries (also known as pressure ulcers) are fundamental aspects of the management of the patient following fragility fracture, especially following hip fracture and associated surgery. Ageing skin and multiple comorbidities are significant factors in skin injury and wound healing problems. The aim of this chapter is to provide the reader with an overview of evidence-based approaches to the prevention of pressure injuries and to wound management following hip fracture surgery.

7.1 Learning Outcomes

At the end of the chapter, and following further study, the nurse will be able to:

- Explain the causes and pathophysiology of pressure injuries
- Recognise risk factors for pressure injury in patients following hip fracture
- Provide evidence-based care to patients at risk of pressure injury
- Discuss the factors that inhibit and enhance wound healing
- Provide evidence-based care to patients with surgical wounds following fragility fracture surgery.

A. Hommel (✉)
Department of Orthopaedics, Skane University Hospital, Malmö, Sweden

Department of Care Science, Malmö University, Malmö, Sweden
e-mail: Ami.hommel@med.lu.se

J. Santy-Tomlinson
Faculty of Biology, Medicine and Health, Division of Nursing, Midwifery and Social Work, School of Health Sciences, The University of Manchester, Manchester, UK
e-mail: Julie.santy-tomlinson@manchester.ac.uk

K. Hertz, J. Santy-Tomlinson (eds.), *Fragility Fracture Nursing*, Perspectives in Nursing Management and Care for Older Adults, https://doi.org/10.1007/978-3-319-76681-2_7

7.2 Pressure Injuries

Pressure injuries are significant breaches of patient safety but are still relatively common following fragility fracture, especially femoral and hip fractures. The term "pressure injury" will be used as it is considered a more accurate term than "pressure ulcer" or "pressure sore" because some presentations are not open ulcers. Pressure injuries result in short- and long-term pain and distress for patients and are often considered indicators of inadequate care quality, leading to litigation. Despite the availability of evidence-based guidelines, nurses' knowledge of pressure injury prevention has been shown to be variable [1]. This is a significant factor in patients acquiring pressure injuries during hospital and care facility admissions as well as in the home care setting. An important part of the process of service improvement to reduce pressure injury incidence is to ensure that practitioners are well educated and possess the skills and knowledge of evidence-based practice in pressure injury prevention.

7.2.1 Pathophysiology and Causes of Pressure Injuries

Pressure injuries are localised areas of soft tissue damage that typically occur in a people who are elderly, have limited mobility or are confined to bed or chair by an acute or chronic health problem, injury or surgery and who have impaired nutrition, as is often the case for patients who are frail and have fragility fractures. These factors mean that the tolerance of the individual's skin and underlying tissues to forces that damage the skin and circulation is reduced. Tissue damage most often occurs when skin and the underlying tissues are subjected to pressure, friction and/or shear or a combination of all three. If pressure, friction or shear are prolonged, they can result in impaired blood supply and damage to skin and underlying tissues [2]. An additional factor in skin injury is moisture, usually from urinary incontinence; if urine is in contact with the skin for prolonged periods, it can lead to incontinence-associated dermatitis (IAD), a type of irritant contact dermatitis caused by prolonged exposure of the skin to urine, faeces [3] or other fluids such as wound exudate and sweat. In combination, pressure, friction, shear and moisture (Fig. 7.1) represent a group of extrinsic factors that healthcare workers need to modify when aiming to prevent skin damage.

In addition to the extrinsic factors discussed above, patients are also vulnerable to tissue injury because of a complex interplay between a variety of intrinsic factors that affect the skin's innate ability to resist external forces—tissue tolerance (Fig. 7.1) [2]. These factors include coexisting health conditions such as those affecting the respiratory and circulatory system which result in diminished blood, oxygen and nutrition supply to the tissues. Pulmonary disease, cardiovascular disease and diabetes are common examples of such conditions. Health conditions that

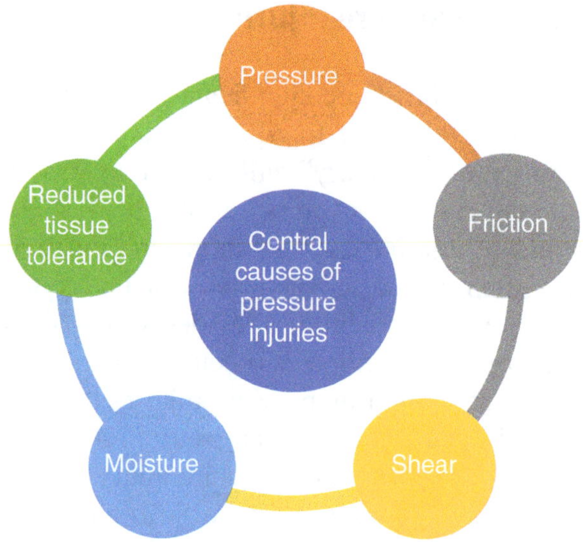

Fig. 7.1 The central causes of pressure injuries

affect mobility such as osteoarthritis and neurological conditions also increase the risk of pressure injury because they restrict the patient's ability to move themselves, mobilise and change their own position in bed or chair.

7.2.2 Classification of Pressure Injuries

Pressure injuries are classified according to the NPUAP/EPUAP/PPIA guidance, updated in 2014 [4]. An understanding of each classification is essential in helping nurses and other staff to recognise the early development of pressure injuries so that deterioration can be prevented. The initial stage of pressure injury is usually redness of the skin, erythema, particularly over bony prominences. In the first instance, this redness indicates an area of skin that has been subjected to pressure and other forces, resulting in an inflammatory reaction that causes local dilation of blood vessels. This is called "blanching" erythema if all redness disappears when light finger pressure is applied, indicating that the local capillaries are undamaged. The patient may state that there is localised pain over a bony prominence even before erythema begins [5]. Blanching erythema is a sign that the patient's position needs to be changed as there is potential for capillary damage if pressure is not relieved. Blanchable erythema is not considered a pressure injury but an important warning sign that preventive measures are needed. If, however, the forces are not removed, blanching erythema can quickly develop into a pressure injury as indicated by category 1 in Box 7.1, non-blanchable erythema of intact skin. Each of the further categories of pressure injury indicates further tissue damage and is much more difficult to reverse than non-blanchable erythema.

Box 7.1: NPUAP/EPUAP/PPIA Classifications of Pressure Injury [4]

Category 1 Pressure Injury: Non-blanchable erythema of intact skin

Intact skin with a localised area of non-blanchable erythema. This may appear differently in darkly pigmented skin. Presence of blanchable erythema or changes in sensation, temperature or firmness may precede visual changes. Colour changes do not include purple or maroon discoloration; these may indicate *deep tissue injury*.

Category 2 Pressure Injury: Partial-thickness loss of skin with exposed dermis

The wound bed is viable, pink or red and moist and may also present as an intact or ruptured serum-filled blister. Adipose (fat) is not visible and deeper tissues are not visible. Granulation tissue, slough and eschar are not present. These injuries commonly result from adverse microclimate and shear in the skin over the pelvis and shear in the heel. This stage should not be used to describe moisture-associated skin damage (MASD) including incontinence-associated dermatitis (IAD), intertriginous dermatitis (ITD), medical adhesive-related skin injury (MARS) or traumatic wounds (skin tears, burns, abrasions).

Category 3 Pressure Injury: Full-thickness skin loss

Full-thickness loss of skin, in which adipose (fat) is visible in the ulcer and granulation tissue and epibole (rolled wound edges) are often present. Slough and/or eschar may be visible. The depth of tissue damage varies by anatomical location; areas of significant adiposity can develop deep wounds. Undermining and tunnelling may occur. Fascia, muscle, tendon, ligament, cartilage and/or bone is not exposed. If slough or eschar obscures the extent of tissue loss, this is an *unstageable pressure injury*.

Category 4 Pressure Injury: Full-thickness skin and tissue loss

Full-thickness skin and tissue loss with exposed or directly palpable fascia, muscle, tendon, ligament, cartilage or bone in the ulcer. Slough and/or eschar may be visible. Epibole (rolled edges), undermining and/or tunnelling often occur. Depth varies by anatomical location. If slough or eschar obscures the extent of tissue loss, this is an *unstageable pressure injury*.

7.2.3 Pressure Injury Prevention

Interventions to prevent pressure injuries must be led by the latest evidence-based guidance and coordinated by the multidisciplinary team. The NPUAP/EPUAP/PPPIA guidelines [4] provide direction for practice across the world and the following advice is based on this guidance. The implementation of guidance, evaluation of practice and regular audit and monitoring of pressure injury prevalence or incidence should be led by local experts with responsibility for service improvement [6]. This should include reporting, investigation and cause analysis of hospital- and care facility-acquired pressure injuries.

7.2.3.1 Patient Assessment

Assessment of the patient is central to planning effective preventive care as it provides an understanding of the risk factors which can be mitigated by effective evidence-based care. The ongoing assessment of the patient should include:

- Full skin assessment as soon as possible (but within 8 h) after admission and thereafter at least daily, or more frequently if the patient's health deteriorates or healthcare interventions such as procedures or surgery increase the risk of pressure injury.
- Inspection should focus on common pressure points over bony prominences such as the sacrum, buttocks, heels, the back of the head, elbows, shoulders, hips (over the greater trochanter), ischial tuberosities, sides of knees and ankles/malleoli.
- Assessment should also include taking note of any medical and other devices (e.g. casts, urinary catheters, intravenous lines, oxygen masks, straps and ties) that can lead to additional pressure points.
- Skin inspection should note any broken, discoloured, dry/flaking, papery (thin/fragile), clammy, oedematous (puffy) or mottled skin: all of which increase the risk of, or indicate the existence of, tissue injury. Any red or discoloured skin over bony prominences indicates possible tissue damage and must be acted upon immediately to prevent deterioration.
- A structured risk assessment should be carried out as soon as possible (but within 8 h) after admission to identify any risk of pressure injury development and the individual factors that require intervention. Patient characteristics that indicates potential risk of pressure injury should be documented in the risk assessment including; patient age, medical conditions impacting on tissue health and drug or other therapy impacting on tissue health. Risk assessment is not, however, an end in itself and it is important that it then leads to active intervention to modify the risk factors.
- Any existing or new pressure injuries should be recorded and classified according to the NPUAP/EPUAP/PPPIA classification system [4] in Box 7.1.

It must be stressed that assessment alone is not sufficient to reduce the incidence of pressure injuries [7] and that it is the preventive interventions that follow that are the most important actions to be taken.

7.2.3.2 Evidence-Based Preventive Interventions

Pressure injury prevention must be a priority for the whole clinical team but tends to be led by the nursing team. Pressure injuries are important indicators of the quality of nursing care and the development of an avoidable injury is a breach in patient safety. Assessment and interventions for prevention and treatment of pressure injuries need to be patient-centred. Although much research has been conducted into the causes of and most effective methods of prevention and there is much evidence-based guidance readily available, pressure injuries are still a significant problem for hospitalised patients [8]. The local, national and international incidence of hospital-acquired pressure injuries is difficult to quantify, but they are often the largest proportion of patient safety incidents and failures in prevention that lead to hospital-acquired pressure injuries can be viewed as healthcare-associated complications and are sometimes considered an indicator for the quality of nursing. The results of a European prevalence study, in 2002, suggested that as few as 10% of patients at risk of pressure injuries were receiving enough preventive care [9].

The UK National Health Service [10] has developed an approach to pressure injury prevention known by the acronym S.S.K.I.N. (Skin, Surface, Keep moving, Incontinence and Nutrition) which provides a useful approach to identifying evidence-based interventions for the prevention of pressure injuries as follows:

Skin: Fundamental care that helps to maintain the skin's protective purpose includes keeping the skin clean and dry using unscented skin cleansers that do not cause irritation. This is particularly important for patients with older, dry skin and for those with skin allergies and other skin conditions. It is also helpful to protect the skin's moisture barrier by regularly applying a light layer of simple, unscented moisturisers or emollients while avoiding the overuse of creams and lotions. Positioning the patient on areas of erythematous (red) skin and massaging the skin should be avoided. Massage causes friction and shear that can damage the delicate microcirculation and lead to inflammation and tissue damage.

Surface: Support surfaces on both beds and chairs should meet individual patient needs as well as operating tables during surgery. Support surface choice is based on the patient's level of mobility; those who are largely bedbound (e.g. while awaiting surgery or immediately afterwards) may benefit from the use of an alternating pressure mattress, but this should never replace the need for repositioning (see keep moving below). The relative merits of these higher specification support surfaces in preventing pressure injuries are unclear [11]. Once the patient can sit out of bed, it is essential that risk of pressure injuries is still acknowledged and a pressure redistributing cushion is used until the patient is fully mobile.

Keep moving: The aim of care should be to support remobilisation as early as possible while recognising the effects of reduced mobility during the rehabilitation phase (Chap. 6). Prolonged pressure to bony prominences and other vulnerable areas, along with friction and shear, must be avoided by regular repositioning of the patient, especially if they cannot do this for themselves or mobility is restricted. Good manual handling practice is essential in avoiding friction and shear and heels should be lifted free of the bed surface using pillows. The frequency of repositioning should be based on individual patient need relating to their skin tolerance to pressure (e.g. development of areas of blanching hyperaemia) and their general condition and comfort. Pressure should be relieved or redistributed, and repositioning onto bony prominences should be avoided by using the 30-degree tilt options and profiling bed functions. Once patients can sit in a chair, repositioning should be carried out regularly by encouraging patients to stand, mobilise and return to lying positions depending on frequent skin reassessment.

Incontinence: Incontinence of urine and/or faeces exposes the skin to excessive moisture which can damage the dermal and epidermal cells. Urine, faeces, sweat and exudate contain chemical substances which are toxic to skin cells and can lead to incontinence-associated dermatitis [3]. Patients with incontinence should have an individual continence management plan that includes immediate cleansing of the skin following incontinence and the light use of barrier creams to protect the skin. The absorbency of continence products such as pads can be affected by barrier creams transferred from the skin to the pad.

Nutrition: Nutritional assessment and screening should be conducted to identify patients who are malnourished or at risk of malnourishment. It is essential to ensure that there is an adequate supply of nutrients—particularly protein, energy, water and vitamins—to the skin. An individualised nutrition plan is needed for anyone with or at risk of malnutrition (see Chap. 9 for further information).

7.3 Wound Management

Because the definitive management of hip fracture, and some other fragility fractures that require surgical fixation, almost always involves surgery (see Chap. 5), most patients require acute wound care during the hospital stay and following discharge. Surgical wounds are an important source of potential complications due to risk of infection, haematoma and wound healing problems such as dehiscence.

Surgical wounds occur under controlled circumstances and surgeons endeavour to ensure minimal tissue loss and good approximation of the wound edges during wound closure. The main aim of care of the wound is that it should heal rapidly without complications such as infection or dehiscence (breakdown). However, for many patients who have surgery following fragility fracture, their general health is poor and they have multiple pre-existing health problems and medications which can significantly affect healing. It has been reported that occurrence of deep infection following surgery for hip fracture is between 1.5% and 7.3% depending on comorbidities [12]. Understanding the factors that can lead to poor healing and, particularly, surgical site infection as well as the best methods to facilitate healing and prevent infection are important nursing activities both in the pre- and post-operative period as, even preoperatively, a well-prepared patient can make a significant difference to avoiding surgical complications and their consequences.

Wound healing is the process by which function to damaged tissue is restored following surgery. It is a dynamic, complex process that is significantly affected by the nature of the wound, pre- and post-operative management, the patient's health status, the care environment and the care given. Some surgical wounds may be considered a straightforward interruption in the continuity of the protection by the skin resulting from surgery that can be expected to make rapid and predictable progress towards healing [13]. For the older person who has undergone surgery, however, there are numerous factors which place the wound at greater risk of wound healing problems such as infection, haematoma and dehiscence as well as sepsis and death. To facilitate optimal wound healing, the general health and well-being of the patient must be optimised both pre- and post-operatively while considering the patient's past medical/surgical history, medications/polypharmacy and current health history as discussed in Chap. 4. Good nutrition (see Chap. 8) is also central to ensuring wound healing without complications especially given the prevalence of malnutrition in elderly hospitalised patients who may have undergone lengthy periods of fasting preoperatively.

7.3.1 Preventing Wound Infection

Orthopaedic surgery results in a wound that penetrates through all layers of soft tissue to bones and joints making infection a significant worry as deep surgical site infection can lead to implant site infection (where there has been a need for surgical fracture fixation or hemi- or total arthroplasty), osteomyelitis and wound dehiscence, resulting in pain and discomfort, poor outcomes from surgery and delayed discharge.

The use of the most recent evidence-based guidelines [14] for preventing hospital-acquired infections (HAIs) is central to the prevention of surgical site infection. Such guidelines tend to focus on the following important interventions which should be employed for all patients following fragility fracture and surgery:

- Careful attention to hand hygiene
- Hospital environmental hygiene

Specific measures for the prevention of surgical site infection should also be employed [13] including:

- Careful preoperative preparation and perioperative care including skin preparation and antibiotic prophylaxis according to national and international evidence-based guidance and medical team instructions
- Ensuring the patient's general health status and tissue perfusion is optimised through good nutrition and hydration
- Stringent aseptic technique when caring for wounds and removing and handling wound drains
- Removing wound drains as soon as possible, if possible within 24 h of surgery
- Covering wounds with an appropriate sterile dressing until it is evident that the initial stages of wound healing have been completed and the wound surface is, at least, superficially sealed
- Removing the dressing and disturbing the wound as little as possible; dressings should only be removed and replaced if there are signs that there has been "strike through" (blood or exudate has soaked through the dressing) or the wound needs inspection because of pain and other symptoms of infection
- Where wound closure materials (e.g. sutures or staples) need removal, this should be done at the appropriate time (when healing is anticipated) and only following careful inspection of the wound; wound closure materials should not be left in for longer than necessary
- Any identified problems with the wound should be reported immediately to the medical team; immediate medical attention is needed if infection is suspected and appropriate antibiotics should then be prescribed

- Assessment and surveillance of the wound in the post-operative period for signs of infection (wound breakdown (dehiscence) pain, particularly that which is increasing, redness and wound discharge) until recovery is complete; in wounds that involve orthopaedic implants, infection may appear any time up to 1 year after surgery
- Laboratory analysis of wound samples such as swabs can be useful in providing information about what organisms may be colonising the surface of the skin but is not helpful in diagnosing deep infection unless there is wound discharge. Hence, wound samples should only be taken of discharging exudate.

7.4 Summary of Key Points for Learning

An understanding of the pathophysiology of pressure injuries by nurses is a fundamental aspect of pressure injury prevention. Nurses need to be able to recognise the risk factors for pressure injury, including red skin, particularly in patients who are at elevated risk, such as those with hip fracture. Evidence-based care should include a focus on skin assessment, support surfaces, keeping the patient moving by ensuring mobility and/or frequent changes of position, ensuring good nutrition and hydration and effectively managing skin moisture, especially relating to incontinence.

The effective evidence-based management of surgical wounds following surgery after fragility fracture can be challenging as ageing and comorbidities affect wound healing. Wound care involves careful wound assessment and observation and attention to infection prevention measures while managing the factors that affect wound healing for individual patients.

7.5 Suggested Further Study

- Download the National Pressure Ulcer Advisory Panel, European Pressure Ulcer Advisory Panel and Pan Pacific Pressure Injury Alliance (NPUAP/EPUAP/PPPIA) (2014) Prevention and Treatment of Pressure Ulcers: Quick Reference Guide. From: http://www.epuap.org/wp-content/uploads/2016/10/quick-reference-guide-digital-npuap-epuap-pppia-jan2016.pdf. Identify someone in your team who might be a good person to act as a champion for ensuring the guidelines are implemented in your clinical area (this might, of course, be you or you can support them). Discuss with them which aspects of the guidelines your unit achieves least well or that you feel are the most important to tackle. Discuss how you might approach changing one area of practice to ensure you meet the guidelines.
- Find out where you can access data about wound infection rates (1) nationally and (2) in your unit. How does your unit compare to the national rates? Think about how surgical wound care is practised in your unit compared to the recommendations presented in this chapter. Write a reflection that includes recommendations for at least one improvement in practice and develop an action plan.

References

1. Gunningberg L et al (2013) Pressure ulcer knowledge of registered nurses, assistant nurses and student nurses: a descriptive, comparative multicentre study in Sweden. Int Wound J 12:462. https://doi.org/10.1111/iwj.12138
2. NICE (2014) Pressure ulcers: prevention and management. Clinical guideline, vol 179. www.nice.org.uk/guidance/cg179
3. Beeckman D (2017) A decade of research on incontinence-associated dermatitis (IAD): evidence, knowledge gaps and next steps. J Tissue Viability 26:47–56
4. National Pressure Ulcer Advisory Panel, European Pressure Ulcer Advisory Panel and Pan Pacific Pressure Injury Alliance (NPUAP/EPUAP/PPPIA) (2014) Prevention and Treatment of Pressure Ulcers: Quick Reference Guide. In: Haesler E (ed) Cambridge Media: Osborne Park, Australia. http://www.epuap.org/wp-content/uploads/2016/10/quick-reference-guide-digital-npuap-epuap-pppia-jan2016.pdf
5. Smith I et al (2017) Exploring the role of pain as an early predictor of pressure ulcers: a prospective cohort study. BMJ Open 7:e013623. https://doi.org/10.1136/bmjopen-2016-013623
6. Hommel A et al (2017) Successful factors to prevent pressure ulcers—an interview study. J Clin Nurs 26:182–189. https://doi.org/10.1111/jocn.13465
7. Moore Z, Cowman S (2014) Risk assessment tools for the prevention of pressure ulcers. Cochrane Database Syst Rev (2):CD006471. https://doi.org/10.1002/14651858.CD006471.pub3
8. Sving E et al (2014) Factors contributing to evidence-based pressure ulcer prevention. A cross-sectional study. Int J Nurs Stud 51:717–725
9. Vanderwee K et al (2007) Pressure ulcer prevalence in Europe: a pilot study. J Eval Clin Pract 13(2):227–235
10. NHS (2016) Stop the pressure. Helping to prevent pressure ulcers. NHS Improvement. http://nhs.stopthepressure.co.uk/
11. McInnes E et al (2011) Support surfaces for pressure ulcer prevention. Cochrane Database Syst Rev (4):CD001735. https://doi.org/10.1002/14651858.CD001735.pub4
12. de Jong L et al (2017) Factors affecting the rate of surgical site infection in patients after hemiarthroplasty of the hip following a fracture of the neck of the femur. Bone Joint J 99-B:1088–1094. https://doi.org/10.1302/0301-620X.99B8
13. Donnelly J et al (2014) Wound management, tissue viability and infection. In: Clarke S, Santy-Tomlinson J (eds) Orthopaedic and Trauma Nursing. An evidence based approach. Wiley/Blackwell, Oxford
14. Loveday H et al (2014) epic3: National evidence-based guidelines for preventing healthcare associated infections in NHS hospitals in England. J Hosp Infect 86(Suppl 1):S1–S70. https://doi.org/10.1016/S0195-6701(13)60012-2
15. Coleman S et al (2014) A new pressure ulcer conceptual framework. J Adv Nurs 70(10):2222–2234

Nutrition and Hydration

8

Patrick Roigk

Malnutrition and dehydration are important aspects of the care of older people, particularly those in hospitals or in long-term care facilities. Many older people do not eat and drink adequately during hospital stays and, following hip fracture, many patients achieve only a half of their recommended daily energy, protein and other nutritional requirements [1]. This leads to poor recovery and diminished health status and functional ability and results in a higher risk of other complications (Chap. 6).

Nurses are the coordinators of the care process, so it is essential that they bring other health-care specialists together as a team to collaboratively provide high-quality care that reflects patients' needs for assessment, intervention and health promotion. When an interdisciplinary team (orthogeriatric collaboration) work together care is more successful, improves patient outcomes and reduces the risk of the in-hospital and long-term mortality.

The aim of this chapter is to increase awareness of nurses' responsibility, within a multidisciplinary team, for assessment and intervention of nutrition and hydration, examine the issues pertaining to nutrition and fluid balance in older people and outline the nature, assessment and interventions relating to malnutrition and dehydration.

8.1 Learning Outcomes

At the end of the chapter, and following further study, the nurse will be able to:

P. Roigk
Department of Clinical Gerontology and Rehabilitation, Robert-Bosch-Hospital, Stuttgart, Germany
e-mail: Patrick.roigk@rbk.de

K. Hertz, J. Santy-Tomlinson (eds.), *Fragility Fracture Nursing*, Perspectives in Nursing Management and Care for Older Adults, https://doi.org/10.1007/978-3-319-76681-2_8

- Identify those at risk of malnutrition and dehydration
- Prevent complications of poor nutrition and dehydration through effective intervention and health promotion
- Identify the nurse's role in coordination of the interdisciplinary team to best meet patients' needs.

8.2 Healthy Diet for Older Adults

In developed countries, people are currently consuming more food high in energy, fats, sugars and salt than in previous decades. While undernutrition leads to a higher risk for health problems, obesity also increases morbidity and mortality from diabetes, hypertension and cardiovascular diseases. To change unhealthy behaviour, education about healthy lifestyles is necessary. A healthy diet prevents malnutrition in every form. A healthy diet for adults contains [2]:

- At least 400 g (5 portions) of fruit and vegetables a day
- Less than 10% of total energy intake from free sugars (equivalent to 50 g for a person of healthy body weight consuming approximately 2000 calories per day)
- Less than 30% of total energy intake from fats; unsaturated fats (e.g. fish, avocado, nuts, olive oil) are preferable to saturated fats (e.g. in fatty meat, butter, palm and coconut oil)
- Less than 5 g of salt per day and use iodised salt.

The recommended daily fluid intake for people over the age of 65 years is 2250 ml. This consists of approximately 60% direct fluid (from drinking) and approximately 40% of indirect fluid (from food and oxidation) [3]. In the case of kidney or heart diseases or other health problem that necessitates restriction of fluid intake, a physician should be involved in calculating the appropriate amount of daily fluid required. Older people, especially those recovering from fracture and surgery, have fluctuating metabolic needs and health practitioners must ensure that sufficient energy and other nutrients are available for recovery and wound healing.

With increasing age, physiological and psychological changes increase the incidence of chronic diseases, fractures and disabilities due to the changing metabolism and lack of knowledge of individuals about appropriate strategies to prevent malnutrition [4]. While the requirement of nutrition (e.g. carbohydrates and fats) decreases with older age, the requirement of vitamins and minerals is stable [5]. Most patients in hospitals are over the age of 60 years. Therefore, it is essential that they have a diet with less energy but rich in nutrition and that this is altered to a diet higher in energy when they are ill or recovering from fractures and surgery. This decreases the risk of falls, fractures and osteoporosis and supports recovery and healing.

Table 8.1 Dietary sources of calcium

Main sources of calcium (250 mg)	Additional sources of calcium (100 mg)
200 ml milk	100 g broccoli
180 g yoghurt	100 g leguminous plants (dry weight)
30 g hard cheese	300 g granary bread
60 g soft cheese	40 g almonds
200–250 g curd	25 ml calcium rich mineral water

Nurses must be aware of this baseline information so that they can educate patients and carers about healthy eating and fluid intake. If patients need more detailed support with their individual nutrition status, other members of the interdisciplinary team should be involved, such as dieticians, and written resources provided.

8.3 Calcium and Vitamin D

Two crucial factors in bone health are calcium and vitamin D; vitamin D is essential for the uptake and absorption of calcium. The recommended daily amount of calcium for people over 65 years is 1000 mg [6]. Table 8.1 shows the main sources of calcium with minimum amounts of 250 mg and 100 mg calcium, which should be a regular part of meals to meet the needs.

Vitamin D is a fat-soluble vitamin which is important for calcium uptake in bones, especially in later life. Food contains small amounts of vitamin D, but the production of vitamin D takes place in the skin under the influence of ultraviolet (UV) light. Production of vitamin D is limited where sunshine is depleted, e.g. in northern Europe and northern North America, particularly in winter. The capacity to produce vitamin D decreases in older age by four times, resulting in lower levels of vitamin D [7]. It is recommended to expose the hands, arms and face to sunlight for approximately 5–25 min per day, but this is limited during hospitalisation and by other social factors, so supplementation should be prescribed. The recommendation for an adequate supplementation of vitamin D intake for older people is 800–1000 IU per day [8] and it should be taken with main meals [9].

Although nutrition is important in preventing osteoporosis-associated fractures, it is also essential for maintaining the positive effects of weight-bearing activity and exercise training on bone density [10]. Regular physical activity of 30 min per day promotes calcium resorption and supports muscle growth and bone density [11]. Following hip fracture, patients should be encouraged to participate in daily activity as a part of their discharge plan, supported by inpatient or outpatient rehabilitation programmes. If patients are independent in activities of daily living and do not suffer from other health problems or disabilities which limit physical activity, additional information about specific exercises and activities should also be provided.

8.4 Malnutrition and Dehydration

To identify and treat patients with malnutrition or dehydration, nurses must know how malnutrition and dehydration is defined. According to NANDA [12], malnutrition is: 'Intake of nutrients insufficient to meet metabolic needs'. The criteria for malnutrition are [13]:

- Body mass index (BMI) < 18.5 kg/m^2
- Unintended weight loss >10% in the last 3–6 months
- BMI < 20 kg/m^2 and unintended weight loss >5% in the last 3–6 months
- Fasting period >7 days (additional criterion).

The definition of dehydration is more complex as it can refer to both loss of body water and volume depletion following the loss of body water; it is suggested [14] that it is defined as a complex condition resulting a reduction in total body water. This can be related to both total water deficit ('water loss dehydration') and combined water and salt deficit ('salt loss dehydration') due to both too low intake and excessive/unbalanced excretion.

8.4.1 Prevalence

The prevalence of malnutrition in care facilities differs widely depending on location. Especially in geriatric wards, where the prevalence is higher than on coronary wards [15]. The estimated number of patients with malnutrition is approximately 35% with 30–55% admitted to acute hospitals being at risk of malnutrition [16].

The reported prevalence of dehydration also varies and depends on which definition of dehydration and which research methods are used. It is estimated that 40% of people newly admitted to hospital are dehydrated and 42% of patients who were not dehydrated at admission were dehydrated 48 h later. Because people who live in residential institutions are very frail, dehydration is estimated to be 46% in these settings [14].

8.4.2 Symptoms of Malnutrition and Dehydration

The symptoms of malnutrition vary and may manifest as weight loss, low energy levels, lethargy, low mood and depression, abdominal cramps or abdominal pain, diarrhoea, limited/reduced muscle tone (sarcopenia) and/or lack of interest in or aversion to eating/drinking.

The signs of dehydration are seen earlier than malnutrition; common symptoms include increasing heart rate, diminished urine output, nausea, dry lips, spasm, unexplained mental confusion [17] and, sometimes, pale mucosa [18].

8.4.3 Screening and Assessing Patients for Malnutrition

Of the range of validated screening and assessment instruments that exist, few have been shown to be valid and reliable including the 3-minute nutrition screening (3MinNS), the Nutritional Risk Screening 2002 (NRS-2002), the Mini Nutritional Assessment (MNA), the Malnutrition Universal Screening Tool (MUST), the Malnutrition Screening Tool (MST—cut off >2) and unwanted weight loss (more than 5% in the last 6 months) [19, 20]. The selection of an appropriate and validated screening instrument should be made according to the patient setting and with common underlying health issues in mind, and multidisciplinary teams need to decide on the best tool for their specific setting.

It is important that the identification and collection of information about people at risk of malnutrition follow two steps:

1. *Screen* all patients within 24 h of admission to identify risk factors for malnutrition.
2. *Assess* all patients at risk for a comprehensive understanding of the problem to enable planning of appropriate interventions.

The risk factors for malnutrition vary between clinical settings and patient groups. Table 8.2 lists common risk factors relating to general and setting-specific factors [21]:

Table 8.2 Main risk factors for malnutrition [21]

General factors	Specific risk factors
Due to illness, therapy and age-related limitations	Hospital
• Acute and chronic illness • Multimorbidity • Side effects of medication • Cognitive impairment • Functional decline • Dysphagia and other eating difficulties	• Illness that affects food intake (e.g. major abdominal surgery) • Fear of diagnosis • Unusual environment • Aversion to hospital food • Interruption of mealtimes
Due to psychosocial limitations	Outpatient care
• Depression • Loneliness and social isolation • Socioeconomic problems • Fears and anxieties • Anorexia	• Limitation on food supply • Limitation to leading an independent life • Limitation to eat independently • Social isolation, loneliness, depression
Due to the environment	Long-term care
• Inflexible mealtimes • Inappropriate help • Disturbance during mealtimes • Unmet need for support	• Interference from the surroundings • Disturbance from other residents • Shame • Wishes not expressed • Aversion to meals and beverages

If there is at risk of malnutrition, the information obtained from screening and assessment should be used to achieve a comprehensive understanding of the individual issues as part of the CGA process to facilitate an individualised plan for avoiding or treating malnutrition. This should include:

- Involvement of family and carers to understand the patient's normal nutritional status and needs.
- Collaboration with members of the interdisciplinary team such as dieticians, physicians, dentists or occupational therapists.
- Discussion with patients, family and carers about the assessment and intervention plans. In case of end-of-life care, the application of artificial nutrition should be discussed in respect of the principles of Bioethics including beneficence, non-maleficence and justice with full consultation the patient, his relatives and the interdisciplinary team.
- Ensure the further treatment of the problem within the discharge management.

8.4.4 Evidence-Based Interventions to Prevent and to Treat Malnutrition

Malnourishment or risk of malnutrition should be approached as a multifactorial problem. It is important that interventions to prevent malnutrition begin with recording a nutrition history and monitoring the patient's food intake during the first days after admission. The treatment of malnutrition can be divided into several specific aspects:

Arrangements for food and meals: Meals in hospitals, and particularly in long-term care facilities, are often tasteless. To improve the taste, nurses should liaise with those responsible for the cooking of meals. Changes in the nature and variety of food or the use of flavoursome sauces are simple and cheap ways to improve taste. As well as the usual timed meals, snacks should be offered by staff or, as self-service, made easily accessible for patients over 24 h. Food should reflect the patient's preferences. For those with physical or psychological difficulties with eating, nurses should assist with the use of appropriate aids (e.g. large handles on cutlery, coloured glasses for visually impaired patients) to help increase independence. Where there are specific problems such as difficulty swallowing or poor dentition, other professionals should be involved as physicians, speech therapists and dentists to address the problem [22].

Dietary supplements: Patients with difficulty eating adequate amounts of food should be offered multi-nutrition supplements with high-protein content (0.9 to 1.2 g/kg/day). Dietary supplements (enteral nutrition) are liquid foods that are used to improve nutritional intake [23]. This is particularly important in frail older people in the perioperative period as there is evidence that dietary supplements, especially for older patients with hip fractures, have a positive effect on quality of life and help to reduce complications [24–26]. To support muscle strength gain during recovery and rehabilitation, high-protein supplements should be combined with muscle resistance training exercise with the physiotherapy team. Patients should be informed about the reason for supplementation and be asked about their preferences in the taste or temperature of the supplement. If patients have intolerances or problems eating and drinking because of the taste, a dietician should be involved. Physicians should be reminded of the need for vitamin D supplementation. Providing information material about healthy diet and fluid intake in older age, particularly about the requirement for minerals and vitamin D, is essential during discharge management.

Interaction during mealtimes: Patients are often highly dependent on the help of nurses, especially those with cognitive or functional decline who are already most at risk of malnutrition, so nurses should consider individual needs for support with eating. Creating a culture in which mealtimes are times of calm with as few interruptions as possible can increase the likelihood that patients eat well [27]. It is also important that enough help is available at mealtimes to support eating and that families are encouraged to be involved.

Environmental and personal requirements: The environment in hospitals and residential facilities can be unfamiliar and impersonal. Mealtimes are important human interaction opportunities normally conducted in pleasant, comfortable surroundings conducive to appetite. Nurses should involve support workers, volunteers and families in creating a pleasant environment for eating, considering issues such as adequate table decoration adapted to the seasons to help patients to be more orientated, feel more comfortable and increase the likelihood of them eating well [28].

Education, support and guidance: Patients and families can be unaware of the problems and the consequences of malnutrition, so education, information, support and guidance are important in engaging patients and carers in eating well. Information needs to be individualised and can be provided in a variety of ways. Some people prefer written information (e.g. leaflets, visual aids or posters), while others prefer technological approaches such as apps on smartphones and/or Internet-based information.

8.4.5 Hydration and Dehydration

Dehydration is common among hospitalised older adults with significant adverse consequences. The screening of those at risk of dehydration is challenging because of the unspecific symptoms and the rapid progress. Box 8.1 lists the main risk factors of dehydration.

8.4.5.1 Screening and Assessing Patients with Dehydration

To identify people at risk of dehydration, nurses should follow the same procedure for the risk of malnutrition. However, unlike malnutrition, there are no validated

Box 8.1: Risk Factors for Dehydration

- Low BMI
- Depleted thirst
- Dependent on care
- Cognitive impairment
- Frailty and comorbidities
- Neurological deficits such as hemi- and paraplegia
- Dysphagia
- Constipation, diarrhoea, vomiting and incontinence
- Fear of incontinence and reluctance to drink
- Taking potassium-sparing diuretics

screening tools, so nurses need to use their knowledge and skills to make individualised assessments by:

1. *Screening* all patients within 24 h of admission to identify risk factors for dehydration.
2. *Assessing* all patients at risk to enable a comprehensive understanding of the problem and a plan of appropriate measures to be devised.

As well as considering the risk factors identified in Box 8.1, criteria for positive risk screening of people for dehydration may include [29]:

- Fatigue and lethargy
- Not drinking between meals
- BIA (bioelectrical impedance analysis) resistance at 50 kHz (BIA assesses electrical impedance through the body commonly from the fingers to the toes and is often used to estimate body fat)

Additional screening tests with limited diagnostic accuracy include:

- Decreasing drink intake
- Diminished urine output
- High urine osmolality
- Low axilla moisture (dry armpits).

8.4.5.2 Assessment and Further Action

If the patient is dehydrated, or at risk of dehydration, screening should achieve a comprehensive understanding of the underlying issues and generate a plan of appropriate measures to treat or prevent dehydration. This should include:

- Close monitoring of both fluid intake and urinary and other fluid output such as vomiting or wound drainage

- Ensure toileting facilities are easily accessible, and if not, or patient's physical activity is limited, use aids such as urine bottles or commodes
- Involvement of the patient and family/carers in the assessment and plan of care, including encouraging fluid intake of approximately 2250 ml per day (direct and indirect fluid) if not contraindicated
- Involvement of other members of the team such as physicians and ensuring that the whole of the nursing team, including support workers/carers, are aware of the risks and the need to closely monitor fluid intake and supplement as required
- Discuss with patients and their family/caregivers the risks, plan of care and aims of care in terms of volume of fluid required and engage family in supporting the aims
- Ensure the problem is included within the discharge plan.

8.4.5.3 Evidence-Based Interventions to Prevent and Treat Dehydration

Patients' oral fluid intake is often inadequate, especially early in the patient pathway while fasting and undergoing perioperative preparation. It is essential to closely monitor and document fluid intake and output and to supplement intake, where necessary, with intravenous fluids.

Prevention aims to ensure the availability of drinks that are pleasant to drink and that patients and families understand for the necessity to drink. Support and help are needed to facilitate adequate intake of oral fluids with the following advice in mind [30]:

Availability of drinks: Drinks should be constantly and easily available. Frequent regular drinks 'rounds' should take place; to support nurses, volunteers or assistants may be given responsibility for this activity. Nursing activities can act as prompts to support patients with drinking oral fluids such as during medication rounds.

Drinking pleasure: Taking pleasure in drinking depends on individual preferences including types of fluid, temperature and flavour. Asking patients/families about preferences and considering factors that can support fluid intake such as reminders to drink and social interaction can be useful.

Support and help to drink: Offering individualised support to patients to help them to drink can encourage adequate fluid intake. This should be done in a friendly, unhurried and calm manner using appropriate drinking aids such as straws and special cups or with bottle-clipped systems. Family often feel helpless but may be able to help with drinking so that they feel involved and useful. Family members can be offered information including how to recognise dehydration and how to help with drinking.

Monitoring and understanding of the necessity to drink: Nurses should provide appropriate information so that patients understand the benefit of adequate fluid intake. Accurately monitoring and recording intake and asking patients/families about the baseline daily fluid intake are essential. All involved need to be aware of the outward signs of dehydration such as:

- Diminished urine output and concentrated urine
- Dry lips, mucous membranes, diminished skin turgor
- Muscle weakness, dizziness, restlessness, headache.

8.5 Summary of Main Points for Learning

- Older people who are hospitalised with a fracture are often overwhelmed and find it difficult to follow a healthy diet and fluid intake.
- The care process begins with screening and monitoring nutritional status and fluid intake of all older people within 24 h of admission.
- To prevent or treat malnutrition or dehydration, the issue should be discussed within the multidisciplinary team to ensure that everyone is aware of the problem and is involved in planning appropriate interventions.
- All patients at risk of malnutrition and dehydration should be assessed to provide a comprehensive understanding of the problem.
- Observation and documentation of nutrition and fluid intake and output should be conducted at least for the first days after admission.
- Patient needs should be discussed with other professions so that appropriate team-based interventions can be planned.
- It is important to involve the patient and family within the care process.
- Appropriate and appealing meals, snacks and drinks for older people should be available and offered with recommended amounts of water, protein, vitamins and minerals (particularly calcium); this should be complemented with supplementary drinks if intake is not adequate.
- The prescription of vitamin D should be discussed with the patient's physician.
- Patient-centred and evidence-based information should be provided and interventions in case of end-of-life care should be appropriate disscused.
- Educating, informing and involving patients and families increases their level of health literacy.
- Malnutrition and/or dehydration management should be included in the discharge plan.

8.6 Suggested Further Study

- Access and read the following review paper. Make some notes about ways in which the paper's conclusions could impact on your practice and that of your team:
  Sauer A et al. (2016) Nurses needed: Identifying malnutrition in hospitalized older adult. NursingPlus Open https://doi.org/10.1016/j.npls.2016.05.001
- Find out what nutritional guidelines are available in your own region. Read them carefully and think about how these could be used, to develop simple strategies for improving diet and fluid intake in your patients and discuss this in your team.
- Undertake an audit of nutrition and fluid charts of patients who are at risk of malnutrition or dehydration. Discuss with the team, including a dietician, whether you are adequately recording intake and output. Reflect on the implications of this has what you could do to improve this practice.

- Develop an information leaflet for patients/families about why and how patients can make sure they get enough to eat and drink. Discuss this within the team.
- Talk with patients/carers/staff about the things they feel that prevent good diet and fluid intake for patients. Reflect on what these conversations suggest about how practice might be developed to improve patient's nutrition and hydration status.

8.7 How to Self-Assess Learning

To identify learning achieved and the need for further study, the following strategies may be helpful:

- Examine local documentation of nursing care regarding nutrition and hydration, and use this to assess your knowledge and performance.
- Seek advice and mentorship from other expert clinicians such as dietician, and seek their help to keep up to date on new evidencc and disseminate to your team.
- Peer review with colleagues can be used to assess individual progress and practice but should not be too formal. There should be open discussion within the team. Weekly case conferences regarding patients with nutrition and hydration problems can identify nurse-focused issues and enable the exchange of expertise. Expertise is conveyed to the various members of the multidisciplinary team by educational initiatives and by fostering a culture where all the patients' problems are considered.
- Seek feedback from colleagues, patients, carers and other members of the team.

References

1. Duncan D et al (2001) Adequacy of oral feeding among elderly patients with hip fracture. Age Ageing 30(Suppl2):22
2. World Health Organization (WHO) (2015) Healthy diet. Factsheet No 394. http://www.who.int/mediacentre/factsheets/fs394/en/
3. Deutsche Gesellschaft für Ernährung e. V. (DGE) German Society for Nutrition (2017) Wasser (Water). http://www.dge.de/wissenschaft/referenzwerte/wasser/
4. EUFIC (European Food Information Council) (2016) New dietary strategies for heathy ageing in Europe (NU-AGE). http://www.eufic.org/en/collaboration/article/new-dietary-strategies-for-healthy-ageing-in-europe
5. Ahmed T, Haboub N (2010) Assessment and management of nutrition in older people and its importance to health. Clin Interv Ageing 5:207–216
6. Warensjo E et al (2011) Dietary calcium intake and risk of fracture and osteoporosis: prospective longitudinal cohort study. BMJ 342:d1473
7. Cashman K et al (2016) Vitamin D deficiency in Europe: pandemic? Am J Clin Nutr 103(4):1033–1044. http://ajcn.nutrition.org/content/103/4/1033.short

8. Dachverband Osteologie e.V. (DVO) (2014) Ossteoporose bei Männern ab dem 60. Lebensjahr und bei postmenopausalen Frauen Leitlinie des Dachverbands der Deutschsprachigen Wissenschaftlichen Osteologischen Gesellschaften e.V. http://www.dv-osteologie.org/uploads/Leitlinie%202014/DVO-Leitlinie%20Osteoporose%202014%20Kurzfassung%20und%20Langfassung%20Version%201a%2012%2001%202016.pdf
9. Mulligan GB, Licata A (2010) Taking vitamin D with the largest meal improves absorption and results in higher serum levels of 25-hydroxyvitamin D. J Bone Miner Res 25(4):928–930
10. National Osteoporosis Foundation (2017) Osteoporosis exercise for strong bones. https://www.nof.org/patients/fracturesfall-prevention/exercisesafe-movement/osteoporosis-exercise-for-strong-bones/
11. Office of the Surgeon General (US) (2004) Bone health and osteoporosis: a report of the surgeon general. 7: lifestyle approaches to promote bone health. https://www.ncbi.nlm.nih.gov/books/NBK45523/
12. NANDA International (2011) Nursing interventions for imbalanced nutrition less than body requirements. http://nanda-nursinginterventions.blogspot.co.uk/2011/05/nursing-interventions-for-imbalanced.html
13. White J et al (2012) Consensus statement: Academy of Nutrition and Dietetics and American Society of Parenteral and Enteral Nutrition. Characteristics recommended for identification and documentation of adult malnutrition (undernutrition). J Parenter Enter Nutr 36(3):275–283. https://doi.org/10.1177/0148607112440285
14. Thomas D et al (2008) Understanding clinical dehydration and its treatment. J Am Dir Assoc 9:292–301
15. Meijers J et al (2008) Malnutrition prevalence in the Netherlands: results of the annual Dutch National Prevalence Measurement of care problems. Br J Nutr 101(3):417–423
16. Barker L et al (2011) Hospital malnutrition: prevalence, identification and impact on patients and the healthcare system. Int J Environ Res Public Health 8:514–527
17. El-Sharkawy AM et al (2014) Hydration in the older hospital patient—is it a problem? Age Ageing 43:i33–i35
18. Hooper L et al (2015) Clinical symptoms, signs and tests for identification of impending and current water-loss dehydration in older people. Cochrane Database Syst Rev (4):CD00964
19. Poulia K et al (2012) Evaluation of the efficacy of six nutritional screening tools to predict malnutrition in the elder. Clin Nutr 31:378–385
20. Lim S et al (2013) Validity and reliability of nutrition screening administered by nurses. Nutr Clin Pract 28(6):730–736
21. DNQP (2017) Expertenstandard Ernährungsmanagement zur Sicherung und Förderung der oralen Ernährung in der Pflege. 1. Aktualisierung. Universität Osnabrück
22. Abbott RA et al (2013) Effectiveness of mealtime interventions on nutritional outcomes for the elderly living in residential care: a systematic review and meta-analysis. Ageing Res Rev 12(4):967–981
23. Nieuwenhuisen W et al (2010) Older adults and patient in need of nutritional support: review of current treatment options and factors for influencing nutritional intake. Clin Nutr 29:160–169
24. Gunnarsson A et al (2009) Does nutritional intervention for patients with hip fractures reduce postoperative complications and improve rehabilitation? J Clin Nurs 18(9):1325–1133
25. Volkert D et al (2006) ESPEN guidelines on enteral nutrition: geriatrics. Clin Nutr 25(2):330–360
26. Milne A et al (2006) Meta-analysis: protein and energy supplementation in older people. Ann Intern Med 144(7):538
27. Young AM et al (2013) Encouraging, assisting and time to EAT: improved nutritional intake for older medical patients receiving protected mealtimes and/or additional nursing feeding assistance. Clin Nutr 32(4):543–549
28. Nijs K et al (2009) Malnutrition and mealtime ambiance in nursing homes. J Am Med Dir Assoc 10(4):226–229

29. Hooper L et al (2015) Clinical symptoms, signs and tests for identification of impending and current water-loss dehydration in older people. Cochrane Database Syst Rev (4):CD009647
30. Godfrey H et al (2012) An exploration of the hydration care of older people: a qualitative study. Int J Nurs Stud 49(10):1200–1211

9 Nursing the Patient with Altered Cognitive Function

Jason Cross

Cognitive syndromes are common in the older surgical patient. This chapter aims to provide an overview of the causes of altered cognitive function, provide advice on strategies that can be used to identify those at risk and give examples of assessments and interventions to aid diagnosis and treatment. The focus will be on acute confusion or "delirium" but will also comment on how existing cognitive impairment, dementia and depression can impact on patient recovery.

9.1 Learning Outcomes

At the end of the chapter, and following further study, the nurse will be able to:

- Identify patients at risk of delirium
- Apply evidence-based tools to assist in the diagnosis and assessment of delirium, depression, cognitive impairment and dementia
- Discuss management strategies and priorities in the patient with delirium, dementia and depression
- Recognise how the ability to give informed consent is impacted by the presence of acute confusional state (delirium) or dementia.

J. Cross
POPS Team (Proactive Care of the Older Person Undergoing Surgery), Guys and St Thomas' NHS Foundation Trust, London, UK
e-mail: Jason.Cross@gstt.nhs.uk

K. Hertz, J. Santy-Tomlinson (eds.), *Fragility Fracture Nursing*, Perspectives in Nursing Management and Care for Older Adults, https://doi.org/10.1007/978-3-319-76681-2_9

9.2 Assessment of Baseline Health: General Comment

To recognise a change in an individual's function, there needs to be a robust general assessment to identify and document baseline level of physical and mental health. Comprehensive geriatric assessment (CGA) is an effective way to undertake such assessment, with an evolving literature base detailing improvements in patient and clinical reported outcomes, when utilising CGA methods in preoperative assessment [1]. CGA is considered in more detail in Chap. 4.

9.3 Delirium

Delirium is terrifying for the patient (with approximately 50% recalling the episode) and distressing for family and care workers. All nurses are familiar with the patient who suddenly becomes agitated, aggressive or "not right". Delirium, sometimes called "acute confusional state", is common and can occur after any surgical procedure, with an incidence of up to 60% after hip fracture. It is categorised by a sudden onset of fluctuating altered consciousness with changes to perception and cognitive function. It is a serious condition that is associated with poor outcomes (see Box 9.1), but it can be prevented and treated with early assessment and intervention [1].

Box 9.1: Consequences of Delirium

- More hospital-associated complications (pressure injuries, falls)
- Increased stay in hospital or high dependency/critical care in hospital
- Increased incidence of dementia
- More likely to require long-term care/support on discharge
- More likely to die in the short and long term

Managing delirium is challenging, especially when the patient is unable to articulate how they are feeling or is resistant to treatment. Interventions are often only implemented after the patient has developed delirium, with the delirium usually an indicator that the patient is acutely unwell. There is rarely one single predictor of delirium, with it often being a multifactorial combination of long-standing and acute factors. This invariably leads to it being poorly recognised and managed, resulting in increased stress and anxiety for patients, relatives and staff faced with the acutely unwell, rapidly deteriorating, delirious patient.

9.3.1 Assessment

Prevention is more effective than a cure, with any intervention needing to begin early. In the surgical setting, this should be done early in the preoperative period.

Table 9.1 Predisposing and precipitating factors for delirium

Predisposing factors	Precipitating factors
• Age • Dementia or cognitive impairment • Depression • History of delirium • Severe illness or hip fracture • Polypharmacy • Malnutrition/dehydration • Functional dependency • Sensory impairment	• Change in environment • Sleep deprivation • Loss of sensory aids/clues • Physical restraints • Constipation • Urinary retention • Sepsis • Acute illness (e.g. MI) • Untreated pain or excess use of analgesics

Assessment can be problematic in emergency/urgent care where time is limited, especially where best practice relies on patients proceeding to surgery as soon as possible. There are "rapid" tools and questions that can assist in identifying those at risk from delirium. Table 9.1 provides a list of predisposing (currently existing) and precipitating (potential causes) for delirium. The prompt recognition of predisposing factors is essential because; (1) many of these factors are modifiable or can be improved and (2) the non-modifiable risk factors raise awareness of the risk of delirium, providing the impetus for interventions.

Cognitive impairment is a predisposing factor for developing delirium and all patients must have cognitive screening on admission to help identify risk. Assessment starts with simple questions such as asking the patient if they have noticed: "…any change in your memory?". This standard screening, used in both hospital and community settings, should then be supported with a more detailed assessment. There are numerous tools and assessments that highlight cognitive decline, but a simple, practical tool to identify those at risk, with one to two more detailed cognitive screening assessment tools to help further assess cognitive deficits and allow onward care planning, is needed.

The "4AT": The 4AT is a brief, easy-to-use, validated tool used to assess for the presence of delirium and identify moderate to severe cognitive impairment [2] with little training needed. It is sometimes preferred to the "abbreviated mental test score" (AMTS) and is free to use and download (www.the4at.com). It can be used for both initial screening and a daily assessment tool to monitor delirium and allows testing of patients with severe drowsiness or agitation. There are four sections with a score for each answer:

1. *Alertness*: How awake are they? Are they easily woken?
2. *AMT4*: An abbreviated version of the AMT, asking the patient to recall their location, date of birth and age and to state the current year.
3. *Attention*: Asked to list the months of the year backwards.
4. *Acute change or fluctuating course*: Has the patient experienced any hallucinations, paranoia or been acting strangely or "not quite right"?

The more information about baseline cognitive and physical function gathered, the better. A comment made by a family member can provide key information, confirming individual risk factors and helping plan individualised interventions. Families may not recognise the subtle changes in cognition that can signify evolving cognitive decline, so questions should be structured to elicit any deficits in function by, for example, asking if there have been any episodes of confusion or any noticeable decline in memory; who does the shopping and manages the household bills; if able to take medications independently; and if placed in the centre of town, on their own, would they be able to make their way home independently? Deficits in these simple tasks indicate potential cognitive decline.

Performing more detailed cognitive screening may not alter the delirium treatment strategy but can help with detailed planning of ongoing care or referral to specialist teams. There are numerous tools; the following two tests can easily be administered by a nurse with appropriate training:

The Montreal Cognitive Assessment (MoCA): (http://www.mocatest.org/) [3] this tests; visuospatial skill, memory recall and attention, takes about 10 min to complete and gives a total score out of 30; a score of less than 26 indicates cognitive impairment.

The Mini Mental State Examination (MMSE): examines different domains with a score out of 30 indicating cognitive decline. This has a larger evidence base and can differentiate between types of dementia [4]. Used for more in-depth assessment of cognition. Losing favour due to copyright: not free to use. Not as good for mild cognitive impairment.

9.3.2 Identifying Delirium

Delirium is a medical emergency. Early identification is key to managing the confused patient as well as the acute issue that has been the trigger. Attempts to prevent delirium will not always stop it from developing, so there is a need for sensitive vigilance to any change in patients' behaviour.

The "gold standard" assessment and diagnosis of delirium is the Confusion Assessment Method (CAM), a set of four questions that identify whether a patient is delirious. It is well validated and accurate, with a false-positive rate of 10%. Its use by nurses is often poor [5] and education is needed [6]. The CAM relies on nurses to note subtle changes from baseline behaviour; this is often a comment from a colleague or relative noticing an unexpected change in personality or behaviour. The tool should be used as soon as a change in cognition is suspected and repeated at least daily or if the patient's condition changes. The CAM involves four questions (Table 9.2); delirium is confirmed by a "yes" answer to both questions 1 and 2, with a "yes" to either question 3 or 4. Some of the components may fluctuate over time, so it is ideal to question others to ensure a full picture.

9.3.3 Prevention of Delirium

It is feasible to prevent delirium by modifying risk factors using simple single or multicomponent interventions, e.g. correction of an acute kidney injury (dehydration) by giving intravenous fluids or the prescription of analgesia to manage hip

Table 9.2 The Confusion Assessment Method (CAM)

1	*Is there an acute change in mental status from patient's baseline?* • Is there new confusion, agitation, unusual behaviour, hallucinations, paranoia and/or "just not quite right"? • Asking a relative or carer can help with this. *What you may hear:* "After her hip operation my mother became very confused and aggressive. She kept pulling out her drip and shouting at the nurses. It was a shock as she is usually so polite".
2	*Inattention* • Is the patient easily distractible or finding it difficult to follow a conversation? • To help assess this, you can incorporate the months backwards test (see 4AT). *What you may hear:* "I didn't understand what Dad was saying after his operation, one minute he was talking about his knee, and then mentioned being in Germany in the war. Initially I joked with him but he got upset and he was obviously bothered about getting things mixed up".
3	*Disorganised thinking* • May not know where they are or think they are somewhere else • Rambled discussion, jumping from one question to another • Unable to recall the day or time. *What you may hear*: "My wife has mild dementia, but she manages fine at home and we always meet for dinner on Tuesdays. When she was in hospital though, she didn't even recognise me or our daughter; saying we were strangers and there to take her away; it was very upsetting to see".
4	*Altered level of consciousness* • Can be aggressive, shouting, anxious or hyper vigilant • Excessive sleepiness (maybe even unresponsive). *What you may hear:* "My uncle became very confused. He was sleepy at times, and agitated and restless at other times. The nurses gave him medication to help control his symptoms".

pain. Interventions targeting the risk factors for delirium include ensuring the patient has their glasses and hearing aids, maintaining day and night routines, promoting sleep and daytime mobilisation and regularly reorientating patients to time and place. All these strategies, when used in a structured protocol, have been shown to significantly reduce the incidence [7, 8]. It is also essential to communicate with and educate patients and families about the risk of delirium.

9.3.4 Managing the Delirious Patient

Using a tool to identify delirium is only helpful if repeated and supported with detailed assessment of the patient's condition. CAM, for example, will provide a diagnosis but does not provide detail about the severity or expected duration of the episode. Once diagnosed, the patient requires close monitoring and rapid intervention to identify the cause and initiate treatment. A delirious patient will lose capacity to make decisions; this is discussed in the dementia section below. The following four actions should happen within the first 4 h of a diagnosis of delirium:

- *Medical review:* While this requires medical input, many diagnostic interventions can be initiated by the nurse. Figure 9.2 details the causes of delirium with suggested interventions. Many drugs can cause delirium or make it worse.

- *Falls assessment:* Delirious patients are more likely to fall; patients over the age of 65 years having a 30% risk of falling compared to 10% of their non-delirious counterparts [9]. A prompt falls risk assessment should be completed with the emphasis on reducing risk (see Chap. 3). A low bed, bed alarms or enhanced observation should be employed to help maintain a safe environment. In the patient who is agitated and wandering, physical restraint is never appropriate; a patient is more likely to settle if allowed to mobilise with support to maintain safety. The use of bed rails is always discouraged as they act as a barrier that can frighten or agitate the patient further, increasing the risk of them climbing over the rails and falling from a greater height; close monitoring is more effective.
- *Inform family:* Early contact with the patient's family can be the single most effective intervention to assist the healthcare team in the management of the delirious patient. It allows families to feel involved in care, helps reduce stress and provides an opportunity to seek help in managing the delirium. The presence of a relative, friend or carer can be calming, facilitating interventions and relieving the need for close observation by a healthcare team member. This must, though, be done with caution; the presence of a relative with the patient does not reduce the overall risk from delirium, so regular observation and detailed instruction is needed to ensure any change in condition is acted on promptly and appropriately.
- *"HELP" interventions:* Simple multicomponent interventions, or small actions grouped together in a protocol, reduce the symptoms and duration of delirium. The "Hospital Elder Life Program" (HELP) is a system of patient support that aims to maintain cognitive and physical function during hospitalisation and maximise mobility on discharge, helping with discharge and avoiding hospital readmission [10]. Evidence supports the use of HELP, and the protocol focuses on regular monitoring and intervention. The components include:
  - Daily orientation (to time/place)
  - Early mobilisation (maintaining function/normal routine, i.e. using toilet)
  - Feeding assistance (offering regular drinks/helping with feeding)
  - Therapeutic activities (such as board games/playing cards/listening to music)
  - A non-pharmacological sleep protocol (maintaining day/night routine; discouraging daytime sleeping)
  - Hearing/vision adaptations (ensuring hearing and vision aids).

This strategy is only effective if employed alongside regular, at least daily, medical review. Regular or intentional "rounding" using the above components as a checklist can be helpful, the purpose being facilitating interaction and comfort [11].

9.3.5 Medication

A common error in treating delirium is to use antipsychotic medications in excessive doses, give them too late or overuse of benzodiazepines. Sedation in patients with delirium should be avoided and only considered as a last resort if the delirium is posing a significant risk to the patient or others. With proactive early assessment and intervention, patients should not need medication, but if they do, the following should be considered (for guidance only; doses and administration should be based on local evidence-based policy):

- Comprehensive patient medical review: identify causes of delirium that could be treated to alleviate agitation
- Delirium may be superimposed on substance withdrawal and additional pharmacological treatments may be indicated
- ECG (electrocardiogram): medications used to treat delirium can cause changes to heart rhythm
- Haloperidol is the first-line treatment in delirium (exceptions below)
- Lorazepam is first line in patients with delirium who also have Parkinson's disease/parkinsonism, Lewy body dementia or seizures, or if the ECG shows changes.

9.4 Dementia

Dementia is a collective term for a group of degenerative brain diseases including Alzheimer's disease, vascular dementia, Lewy body dementia and frontotemporal dementia. Worldwide, around 50 million people have dementia and there are nearly 10 million new cases every year [12]. The condition has three stages involving increasing deterioration of memory that impacts on functional and emotional health.

Early stage: Often only recognised in retrospect, when the patient enters the middle or later stages of dementia. The person finds it increasingly difficult to concentrate and becomes more forgetful, exhibiting subtle changes in personality, but often remaining independent functionally, although tasks such as managing finances may become difficult.

Middle stage: Unable to retain short-term memory, able to complete basic personal tasks but with reduced safety awareness and may not be able to leave the home alone, usually requiring support to maintain independent living.

Late stage: Withdrawn and requires full care and support, with limited communication and little to no insight into own condition or environment. Motor deterioration is accelerated and may become bed bound; diet may be reduced due to impaired swallow and increased risk of choking; may not eat at all.

At present there is no cure, although some medications can help with the symptoms. As the age of hospital patients increases, more will present with dementia as either a primary (main cause) or secondary condition (as part of background past medical history). Health practitioners must be aware of the impact of dementia on patients, the associated complications and increased risks to health during treatment. Comprehensive history taking is essential in helping to inform and direct care as discussed in the previous section.

Cognitive decline impacts on health and decision-making. Understanding the person's individual needs, desires and feelings can be challenging, leading to significant stress for patients, families and staff in acute care situations. Information must be collected from family or friends, or other health practitioners. Dementia "passports" are documents that can be used to describe the patient, their wants, likes and dislikes - illuminating the patient's personality and providing insight into who the patient is so that care can be planned with an individual's values and beliefs maintained [13]; an example is the "This is me" document [13].

9.4.1 Capacity to Make Decisions

A central aspect of care for all patients with cognitive difficulties is decision-making; be it long term, acute or temporary. Ability to choose what we want and don't want is part of what makes us an individual. To have that ability taken away is distressing and can lead to the values and beliefs of others influencing decisions that may not reflect the individual's own. There are frameworks to help support people with reduced mental capacity in the decision-making process and ensure their best interests are foremost when planning care. In England and Wales, for example, for those over the age of 16, this is the Mental Capacity Act [14], but the following list outlines common principles that help practitioners to best to support patients:

1. Always presume the patient has capacity. They have capacity until proven otherwise.
2. Support people to have capacity through information giving, education and time.
3. People are allowed to make unwise decisions. Not choosing what we perceive as the best course of actions does not indicate a lack of capacity, although may be a sign of reduced understanding.
4. Any treatment must always be in the patient's best interest.
5. If a decision needs to be made without the patient being involved, the least restrictive option should be followed.

Capacity is decision-specific; so when assessing capacity, it is important to know what the question is that requires a decision. For example, it could be a complex decision whether to proceed to surgery or not, involving multiple decisions, or a more simple question regarding taking one medication instead of another. Just because someone may lack capacity regarding one issue, it should not be presumed that this is the same for all issues. If a patient's capacity is in doubt, a two-stage assessment should take place [14]. Box 9.2 is a checklist to make this less daunting.

When an individual who lacks capacity requires treatment, practitioners must ascertain if it is a permanent change in the decision-making process, such as a dementia, or a fluctuating one, such as delirium, drug intoxication or coma. Practitioners must consider what is; (a) in the patient's best interest and (b) the least

Box 9.2: Two-Stage Assessment for Mental Capacity

Stage 1

Should be asked of all patients where concern about capacity is an issue:

- Is there a disturbance of consciousness that could cause the patient to lack capacity (YES or NO)? *For example, is the patient delirious or has known or newly recognised impaired cognition.* If YES—move to stage 2.

Stage 2

Use a four-point capacity test: "can the patient…"

- Understand the information given relevant to the decision, e.g. *information regarding incidence of complication after hip surgery (wound infection, DVT, delirium, success rates* etc.*)?*
- Retain the information given? *Can they repeat back the information given? This only needs to be long enough for the decision to be made.*
- Weigh up or use the information? *Can they discuss the information in context, detailing the pros and cons of the proposed treatment?*
- Communicate their decision? *Can they say what they want to do?*

restrictive option. Practitioners must first ask: can the decision or treatment be delayed to allow time from mental capacity to return? If not, for example, in a time-pressured situation such as surgical fixation following fracture, a best interest decision to ascertain the onward course of care is needed.

9.4.1.1 Advocacy

An advocate can only provide opinion and information; the medical or surgical team can note personal preferences and previous decisions made, but this does give the advocate rights to demand or decline treatments that may be in the best interest of the patient. Anyone can advocate for someone as long as they can confidently; (1) state they know the wants and beliefs of the person who they are advocating for and (2) are not in receipt of financial benefit from their relationship (e.g. a paid carer). When patients cannot make a decision for themselves, it is usually a family member or friend who fulfils the advocate role. In a situation where a family/friend is not available in an emergency situation, the surgical or medical team can proceed anyway, using the information they have at hand to make the 'best interest' decision. In non-emergency situations, where capacity is questioned and unlikely to improve, practitioners can seek the help of an independent mental capacity advocate (IMCA), usually appointed by local authorities and who are charged with the gathering and evaluation of information regarding the views of the individual without capacity and make representations on their behalf. An IMCA should always be sought if the following criteria are met:

- The person is aged 16 or over
- A decision needs to be made about a long-term change in accommodation or serious medical treatment
- The person lacks capacity to make that decision
- There is no independent person, such as a family member or friend, who is "appropriate to consult".

Any best interest "meeting" or discussion must involve as many team members as possible to ensure the decision reached involves aspects that might not be considered by individuals. If all team members cannot be gathered, other forms of communication must be used to ensure all involved are consulted (e.g. via telephone or email) and to ensure all decisions and rationale are documented to provide clarity.

Many countries have human rights legislation that states that all individuals have the right to their liberty being maintained. This can put practitioners in a difficult ethical situation, especially if the patient who lacks capacity resists the treatment being attempted in their best interests, e.g. the "wandering" patient who may try to leave during treatment or the acutely delirious post-operative patient who declines medication. In the UK, for example, the Mental Capacity Act [14] and the Human Rights Act [15] provide guidance on how this can be addressed, providing a framework to legally "deny" the patient without capacity their usual rights to liberty and enforce treatment that is in their best interest. In the UK, an application to apply for a DoLS (Deprivation of Liberty Safeguard) may be instigated through a local government authority, supported by specialist teams. Practitioners should not expect to be able to undertake these comprehensive assessments independently. Once granted, a DoLS can allow restraint and restrictions to keep the patient safe and provide care. Local policies and procedures may differ globally.

9.5 Depression

Everyone gets depressed or down from time to time as a normal reaction to life's difficulties, but clinical depression is different; it is a persistent low mood that affects every aspect of a person's life, leading to social isolation, feelings of worthlessness and, in severe cases, to suicide [16, 17]. The exact cause of clinical depression is not fully understood, although there are recognised risk factors including:

- Personal or family history of depression
- Major life changes, trauma or stress
- Certain physical illnesses and medications.

Depression can occur at any age, but is more likely to develop in adulthood. Simply "being old" does not increase risk of depression, but the accumulation of health issues, along with functional decline and social factors, has been seen to increase the incidence of depression in the older population [18]. Pain, such as chronic back or arthritic pain, is a significant risk factor and, if a diagnosis of depression is already present, can increase the severity of the depressive symptoms [19]. Pain is a factor in reduced function for older people and is under-recognised as a cause of depression. "Aches and pains" are often explained away as normal ageing and the individual may not receive the proactive support needed to break the cycle of pain, leading to worsening low mood, loss of function and isolation [20].

Studies recognise that depression impacts negatively on progress after surgery [17]. The symptoms of clinical depression, such as low motivation, perceptions of non-improvement, sleep disturbance and difficultly with physical rehabilitation, can slow postsurgical recovery [21] with an associated increase in complication rates, with up to 40% of those with anxiety and depression still suffering the effects after discharge [22].

9.5.1 Assessment of Depression

Nurses will often encounter patients with both short- and long-term depression. Clinical assessment and observation should identify existing depression. A comprehensive admission history using alternative sources of information is also essential in highlighting those who may be suffering from depression. In the short term, there may be little that can be done to improve the condition prior to surgery or treatment starting, but assessment can sensitise the team to the risks associated with the depression and allow them to use proactive strategies to help reduce risk. Some of the following will help the practitioner to identify potential for depression [23]:

- History of any mental health disorder
- History of a chronic physical health problem
- Past experience of, and response to, treatments
- Quality of interpersonal relationships
- Living conditions and social isolation
- Family history of mental illness
- History of domestic violence or sexual abuse
- Employment and immigration status.

Nurses can also use an assessment tool to identify those with altered mood, anxiety and depression. There are several tools available, but a simple screening tool will help the practitioner to plan care. Two validated screening tools are recommended by NICE in the UK [24]. These are self-reported questionnaires that give a numerical score; the higher the score, the more likely depression or anxiety will be present:

The Hospital Anxiety and Depression Score (HADS)

Used for initial diagnosis and to track resolution or progression of anxiety and depression. Validated in many languages and for inpatient and outpatient settings; 14 questions with anxiety and depression questions mixed; these are scored separately with a score of 8 or more in either indicating a positive result; takes 2–5 min to complete [25].

The Patient Health Questionnaire 9 (PHQ-9)
More recently developed tool for monitoring and measuring the severity of depression; sometimes used for screening of depression due to its ease of use; score from questionnaire indicates level of depressive symptoms from no symptoms to severe [26].

As patients complete these themselves, it does not add much time to any assessment. However, these assessments should be viewed with caution as patients can exaggerate symptoms, giving false-positive results. The environment where the test is administered can also skew the results, e.g. a person completing the assessment in a room with other people may lead the individual to answer to fit a social expectation [25]. Some tools are copyrighted with cost to reproduce and print.

9.5.2 Interventions

Nurses are well placed to provide the interventions needed to support the patient with depression. Being "at the bedside" provides opportunities to monitor for subtle changes in mood and condition. While the nurse is not expected to be able to perform complex therapeutic techniques, core principles can be integrated into nursing practice. Being caring and compassionate is part of what nurses are, and communication skills and "sixth sense" about potential problems can be an essential component in helping to support patients with anxiety and depression; allowing patients time to talk and express themselves or just letting them be who they are can help build the rapport that can be positive in their recovery.

9.6 Summary of Main Points for Learning

- Cognitive disorders are common and precipitants for delirium/acute confusion
- Delirium is a medical emergency with prompt investigation into its cause essential
- Delirium is related to increased in-hospital and post-discharge morbidity (complications) and mortality (death)
- Early assessment with the addition of a simple tool are essential and key to highlighting those at risk
- A structured approach with simple multicomponent interventions can help reduce delirium and its duration; involving family and carers can be of great benefit
- Capacity should always be assessed when altered cognition is present, i.e. delirium or dementia
- Background information is invaluable in understanding the individuals
- A best interest discussion is useful in helping deciding onward care

- If family or close friend is unable to advocate for a patient with reduced capacity, an independent advocate should be sought
- Any treatment proposed for the patient who lacks capacity should always be the least restrictive option
- Assess early and establish baseline level of needs, both physical and psychological
- Set clear goals for recovery and work with the patient to agree those goals
- Ensure usual psychiatric medications are continued wherever possible
- Consider same staff/team working with the patient to help build rapport
- Reassess depression regularly, allowing time for the patient to discuss their progress, successes and failings.

9.7 Suggested Further Study

- Consider how you do, or could, undertake assessment for cognitive status of your patients. Do an internet search for MMSE (Mini Mental State Examination) and compare this with MoCA. Read more about cognitive assessment using the following resource: http://www.mocatest.org/.
- Examine your national and local guidance about capacity, consent and deprivation of liberties and how this is put into practice where you work. How might this impact on your practice? What should you consider doing differently?
- Examine national guidance about caring for patients with dementia in acute hospital settings.
- Look at self-reported assessment tools that are used, or might be used, to identify patients with depression or anxiety in your area. Could a similar tool be integrated into your practice?

9.8 How to Self-Assess Learning

- Discuss with your clinical team how you might improve the interventions you use to prevent and manage dementia. Could there be more you could implement in your clinical setting? What plans might you put in place for this? Could this become part of "intentional rounding" in your unit?
- What do you understand about the best way to care for patients with delirium and dementia? Discuss this with colleagues and the carers of patients with dementia. How is this reflected in your current practice?

Acknowledgements The support of Dr. Peter Somerville and Guy's and St Thomas' NHS Foundation Trust delirium and dementia (DaD) team, and permission for the use of the guidance referred to in this chapter, was invaluable.

References

1. Partridge JS et al (2017) Randomized clinical trial of comprehensive geriatric assessment and optimization in vascular surgery. Br J Surg 104(6):679–687
2. Bellelli G et al (2014) Validation of the 4AT, a new instrument for rapid delirium screening: a study in 234 hospitalised older people. Age Ageing 3:496–502
3. Nasreddine Z et al (2005) The Montreal Cognitive Assessment, MoCA: a brief screening tool for mild cognitive impairment. J Am Geriatr Soc 53(4):695–699
4. Palmqvist S et al (2009) Practical suggestions on how to differentiate dementia with Lewy bodies from Alzheimer's disease with common cognitive tests. Int J Geriatr Psychiatry 24(12):1405–1412
5. Inouye SK et al (2001) Nurses' recognition of delirium and its symptoms: comparison of nurse and researcher ratings. Arch Intern Med 161:2467–2473
6. Wei LA et al (2008) The confusion assessment method: a systematic review of current usage. J Am Geriatr Soc 56:823–830
7. NICE (National Institute for Health and Clinical Excellence) (2010) Delirium: diagnosis, prevention and management, London. https://www.nice.org.uk/guidance/cg103
8. Marcantonio ER et al (1994) A clinical prediction rule for delirium after elective non-cardiac surgery. JAMA 271(2):134–139
9. Pendlebury S et al (2015) Observational, longitudinal study of delirium in consecutive unselected acute medical admissions: age-specific rates and associated factors, mortality and re-admission. BMJ 5:e007808
10. Inouye SK et al (1999) A multicomponent intervention to prevent delirium in hospitalized older patients. N Engl J Med 340(9):669–676
11. Forde-Johnston C (2014) Intentional rounding: a review of the literature. Nurs Stand 28(32):37–34
12. World Health Organization (2017) Dementia. Fact Sheet. http://www.who.int/mediacentre/factsheets/fs362/en/
13. Alzheimer's Society (2017). This is me—a tool to enable person centred care. https://www.alzheimers.org.uk/download/downloads/id/3423/this_is_me.pdf
14. Mental Capacity Act (2005) London: HMSO
15. Human Rights Act (1998) London: HMSO
16. Richards C et al (2014) The Oxford handbook of depression and comorbidity. Oxford University Press, New York
17. Rosenberger PH et al (2006) Psychosocial factors and surgical outcomes: an evidence-based literature review. J Am Acad Orthop Surg 14(7):397–405
18. Roberts RE et al (1997) Does growing old increase the risk for depression? Am J Psychiatry 154(10):1384–1390
19. Leite AA et al (2011) Comorbidities in patients with osteoarthritis: frequency and impact on pain and physical function. Rev Bras Reumatol 51:118–123
20. Yohannes AM, Caton S (2010) Management of depression in older people with osteoarthritis: A systematic review. Aging Ment Health 14:637–651
21. Block AR et al (2003) The psychology of spine surgery. American Psychological Association, Washington, DC
22. Tully PJ, Baker RA (2012) Depression, anxiety, and cardiac morbidity outcomes after coronary artery bypass surgery: a contemporary and practical review. J Geriatr Cardiol 9(2):197–208
23. Bowling A (2005) Mode of questionnaire administration can have serious effects on data quality. J Public Health 27(3):281–291
24. National Institute for Health and Clinical Excellence (NICE) (2011) Common mental health problems: identification and pathways to care. https://www.nice.org.uk/guidance/cg123
25. Zigmond AS, Snaith RP (1983) The hospital anxiety and depression scale. Acta Psychiatr Scand 67(6):361–370
26. Hunt M et al (2003) Self-report bias and underreporting of depression on the BDI-II. J Pers Assess 80(1):26–23

10 Rehabilitation and Discharge

Silvia Barberi and Lucia Mielli

Fragility fracture is the result of a combination of bone fragility and falls and often leads to hip fracture, a devastating injury for both the patient and their family. The recovery process requires both physical and psychosocial care [1], and much research has focused on physical function, including post-hospital discharge and rehabilitation. All patients presenting with a fragility fracture following a fall should have a full multidisciplinary assessment and interventions to prevent future fractures and falls. The care, rehabilitation and discharge of patients with hip fracture are a significant challenge for many services, but the quality and cost-effectiveness of such care vary considerably. This chapter aims to discuss the role of the nurse in the rehabilitation and hospital discharge phases of the care trajectory.

10.1 Learning Outcomes

At the end of this chapter, and following further study, the nurse will be able to:

- Describe strategies for effective rehabilitation and post-hospital care of older people following fragility fracture
- Describe the role of the nurse in rehabilitation
- Identify and apply strategies for supporting patient motivation and increase self-management during recovery
- Effectively plan patient discharge with the involvement of the patient, family and caregivers.

S. Barberi (✉)
Azienda Ospedaliera San Giovanni Addolorata, Rome, RM, Italy

L. Mielli
Azienda Sanitaria Unica Regionale (ASUR) Marche, Ancona, AN, Italy

K. Hertz, J. Santy-Tomlinson (eds.), *Fragility Fracture Nursing*, Perspectives in Nursing Management and Care for Older Adults, https://doi.org/10.1007/978-3-319-76681-2_10

10.2 Rehabilitation

Following fragility fracture, and especially hip fracture, patients have complex medical, surgical and rehabilitation needs, and social and psychological factors such as fear of falling, self-efficacy, perceived control and coping strategies are important factors in recovery and rehabilitation. Care and rehabilitation of patients following hip fracture are particularly challenging for trauma services, but units that are able to provide good care for these patients will also be able to provide effective care for the complete range of other fragility fractures encountered. The multifactorial nature of the problems facing fragility fracture patients requires a multidisciplinary approach with an emphasis on effective teamwork along with close collaboration between the medical, nursing, physiotherapy, occupational therapy and social care teams. Good multidisciplinary working requires positive attitudes, good communication and sharing of information, an adaptive and flexible approach to collaboration and deep commitment from all concerned to promote quality care and good outcomes for patients.

The primary outcomes of rehabilitation are independence in physical function and quality of life. Poor outcomes of recovery and rehabilitation amount to failure to return to independent living and readmission to hospital. Effective rehabilitation is important in promoting independence and in enabling the patient to reach their potential and return home, as well as minimising costs by reducing the length of hospital stay [2], although there is limited evidence relating to how different care strategies impact on rehabilitation and discharge [3] and there is limited information about who can best provide this care. Early supported multidisciplinary rehabilitation can reduce hospital stay, improve early return to function and impact positively on both readmission rates and the level of public-funded nursing care required.

Increasingly, community rehabilitation schemes are being developed that facilitate early discharge of less frail fracture patients to their own home from the orthopaedic ward. Earlier discharge can be facilitated by referral to a community rehabilitation team, day hospital or other community-based rehabilitation service. Such ongoing rehabilitation allows patients to continue to improve functionally and progress towards their goal after leaving hospital. Collaborative approaches in the acute setting, such as hip fracture programmes [4], can be effective in improving outcomes, and patient rehabilitation and discharge can benefit from intermediate care initiatives such as early supported discharge and care pathways.

10.2.1 Rehabilitation Pathways

From admission, patients should be offered a formal, acute, orthogeriatric or orthopaedic ward-based hip fracture programme that includes all of the following:

- Comprehensive multidisciplinary geriatric/orthogeriatric assessment and continuous review
- Rapid preoperative optimisation of fitness for surgery
- Early identification of individual goals for rehabilitation, to recover mobility and independence and to facilitate return to pre-fracture residence and long-term wellbeing

- Liaison or integration with related services, particularly mental health, falls prevention, bone health, primary care and social services
- Clinical and service governance responsibility for all stages of the pathway of care and rehabilitation, including those aspects delivered in the community.

In many localities, nurses in specialist and advanced roles identify patients suitable for enhanced rehabilitation schemes and ensure their smooth passage through the perioperative period into the rehabilitation phase. After immediate post-operative recovery, it is essential that patients follow a rehabilitation pathway that includes six main elements [3]:

- Assessment of frailty (Chap. 2)
- Establishing goals to maximise mobility and other aspects of function; therapy provided by physiotherapists and occupational therapists has the potential to accelerate the recovery of mobility; the timing of physiotherapy assessment and intervention is important and should begin within 48 h of surgery
- Providing occupational therapy services to assess the need for aids
- Determining strategies to support and improve independence in activities of daily living
- Medication management to ensure all prescribed medications are necessary, the use of antipsychotics and sedatives is minimised and there is effective pain management
- Secondary fracture and fall prevention (Chap. 3).

After hip fracture surgery, patients follow individual pathways through recovery and rehabilitation but, at the same time, patients often experience a common trajectory. "Integrated care pathways" (ICPs) were developed as a way to standardise treatment protocols following hip fracture as well as individualise multidisciplinary management and rehabilitation. These are structured multidisciplinary care plans that describe in detail each step in the process towards rehabilitation and discharge and act as the patient's care record, with the aim of ensuring that the patient receives the recommended standards of care at the appropriate time [5]. Some units have found ICPs helpful in improving key areas of hip fracture care such as optimisation for surgery (often now enshrined in enhanced recovery programmes), early mobilisation, communication with the patient and family, rehabilitation and discharge planning. If such approaches are to be successful as catalysts for high-quality care and rehabilitation, it is essential that all members of the MDT are involved in their development and continuing use.

10.2.2 Mobility and Exercise

As discussed in Chap. 6, mobility and exercise are central to recovery and rehabilitation from injury and surgery. Supported mobility should be an integral part of nursing, using everyday activities such as getting out of bed and walking to the toilet as part of the rehabilitation programme. It is important that this process begins as early as possible after surgery as there is a statistically and clinically significant increase in independence for patients who have early mobilisation compared to delayed mobilisation [6]. Sherrington et al. [7] suggest that exercise programmes should last for at least 2 h a week, for at least 6 months, to reach the desired outcomes.

Mobilisation and other activities need to be reintroduced into patients' activity gradually as their physical recovery from surgery progresses. Important aims include the ability to transfer independently, for example, between a bed and a chair, or ability to rise from a chair [4] as well as walking. When engaged in regularly, these activities can help to improve muscle strength and can impact positively on falls, length of stay, discharge destination, independence in ADLs such as washing and bathing, as well as more complex tasks such as meal preparation. Although this activity should be under the supervision of therapists, it is the nursing team who will most often supervise the patient. Tailored exercises to help improve muscle strength and function should be prescribed by the physiotherapist but supervised by the nursing team and should begin while the patient is in hospital but continued after discharge.

10.2.3 Patient Motivation

The process of rehabilitation involves a transition from one state (helplessness) to another (independence) that needs significant and sustained effort by patients [5]. This process is often described by those who have experienced it as a very difficult event that is fraught with uncertainty, passivity and declining function, needing support in using their inner resources, while they are striving to regain function and independence [8]. To be successful in rehabilitation goals, older people need to be motivated to concord with therapy and exercise programmes and other activities. Social and psychological factors such as fear of falling, self-efficacy and coping strategies are thought to be important in the recovery from hip fracture in older people [9]. Improvements in patient motivation can be achieved by developing a constantly positive approach to patients, with an encouraging attitude and empowering patients to become actively involved in their rehabilitation [10].

Rehabilitation involves major effort from patients. Patient views about their hip fracture and its management and the way they are provided with information are important elements of the natural recovery and treatment process. Caregivers also need information and can influence the recovery process. Patients should receive information and education about the fracture, surgery, risk of future fractures, follow-up and duration of therapy as well as the rehabilitation process. Timely and clear information can reduce stress and uncertainty for patients and potentially improve their outcomes. Caregivers also play a key role in the rehabilitation of elderly patient with hip fracture and can help with motivation, training for walking and facilitation of access to health services, among other aspects. Participation in decision-making, improved access to legal and medical information, possibility of sharing care experiences, presence of a secondary caregiver and increased social support improve the self-efficacy of care, but caregiver overload needs to be carefully considered.

10.3 Discharge and Post-hospital Care

The discharge of an older person from an acute hospital to the most appropriate setting following hip fracture surgery is a complex undertaking requiring careful planning and, if ineffectively conducted, can be the weak link in the passage of the patient from one care setting to another. Premature discharge or discharge to an unsuitable environment can result in hospital readmission. Early hospital discharge may not lead to overall cost-savings if it results in the need for more intense subsequent health-care utilisation, such as ED visits or rehospitalisation. Hospital readmissions are often the result of a fragmented health and social care system [11] and increasing evidence indicates that patients are particularly vulnerable and more likely to experience negative outcomes during these hospital readmissions [12].

Many factors that can increase the likelihood of readmission can be modified so need be considered in the way services are designed and developed. Such factors include; premature discharge, inadequate post-discharge support, insufficient follow-up, therapeutic errors including adverse drug events and other medication-related issues, inadequate transfer handovers and complications of hospital procedures and surgery such as nosocomial infections, pressure ulcers and patient falls.

The patient and family have a right to be involved and supported at every stage of the process so collaboration and continuity of care are central. It is essential that the older person and their family are adequately prepared for discharge, that a care pathway is activated that continues following discharge and that the role of the family and informal carers as partners in the care team is facilitated [13]. Development of a discharge plan must begin as early as possible during the hospital stay, to ensure that patient education and support are provided to facilitate independence and so that the patient can develop an understanding of their health condition and acquire the knowledge and skills needed to self-care independently or with caregiver/family support.

Patients leaving hospital following hip fracture surgery always need further care. To enable discharge, the health-care team must determine the most appropriate setting for ongoing care, considering the continuing care, medical, functional and social needs, and decision-making capacity of the patient. The MDT should collaborate with the patient/family/caregivers and other stakeholders to determine the most suitable plan. Several factors must be considered including; cognitive status, activity level and functional capacity, current home suitability, availability of informal and formal care, availability of transportation and availability of services for ongoing care. The severity of functional impairments and the need for assistance with activities of daily living (ADLs) often determine whether a patient can be safely managed at home or requires care at a skilled nursing facility ("nursing home") or extended care facility ("residential home") with attention to the need for supervision of ADLs and safety awareness.

10.3.1 Discharge Home

For successful discharge home, patients (with help from family or other caregivers, if available) should be able, as a minimum, to:

- Obtain and self-administer medications
- Perform self-care activities
- Eat an appropriate diet or otherwise manage nutritional needs
- Engage with follow-up care.

Availability of appropriate services in the community can influence whether the patient may be safely discharged home. Home services may allow patients who would otherwise need residential care to manage their care needs at home. The lack of a system that ensures continuity of care following discharge home, or other location, can cause serious errors including adverse medication events [14].

10.3.2 Discharge to Another Setting

If discharge home is not appropriate, transfer to another inpatient or residential facility for ongoing care must be arranged. Determining the most appropriate setting for ongoing care involves assessing and matching needs with the capabilities of the potential care setting. One model to help accomplish this involves assessing a set of parameters that describe generic clinical characteristics (medical and surgical issues, mental and emotional status, physical functioning and environment) that are largely independent of the patient's specific diagnosis. These needs are then matched with the services offered at different types of facilities. Once the care team, patient and family have decided that discharge to an alternate facility is necessary, referrals can be made to facilities that are appropriate and meet the patient and family desires and the patient can be screened for acceptance.

Three main types of care facility exist depending on the locality/region/country, each with a different function:

- Acute care hospitals
- Inpatient rehabilitation hospitals, intermediate care/step down units and long-term acute care hospitals
- Nursing and residential care facilities (private or government funded).

Poor information transfer from hospital-based providers to other facilities is common and can contribute to poor discharge/transfer outcomes including the need for readmission, temporary or permanent disability or even death. Discharge information, both written and verbal, should be reviewed with the patient/family and caregivers with an emphasis on assessing and ensuring comprehension. At discharge, the patient should be provided with a document that includes language and literacy-appropriate instructions and patient education materials to help in successful transition from the hospital. These documents should be brief, focused on critical information for the patient and focused on what the patient needs to understand to manage after discharge. One model for patient materials, developed by the National Patient Safety Foundation [15], called "Ask Me 3", includes the following information:

1. What is my main problem? (Why was I in the hospital?)
2. What do I need to do? (How do I manage at home and what should I do if I run into problems?)
3. Why is it important for me to do this?

10.3.3 The Discharge Process

A critical issue leading to discharge problems is lack of planning of the discharge itself. The discharge process must begin on admission to allow time and resources for discharge planning. There are three phases that characterise the discharge process: (1) admission, (2) hospitalisation and (3) discharge.

The admission phase: Within 48 h of admission, the Blaylock Risk Assessment Screening Score (BRASS), a tool that can be used to identify patients who may require a more comprehensive discharge plan, can be used to identify patients at risk of difficult discharge [16] and a referral can be made to the discharge liaison service.

The hospitalisation phase: Once a place of discharge has been decided, contact can be made. If discharge is to be to a continuing care facility (rehabilitation/intermediate care unit or nursing/residential home), individuals involved in the admission to the care facility should visit the patient to assess their suitability for the facility and to discuss this with the patient and family. This visit can enable community care professionals or a continuing care manager to undertake a detailed assessment of the patient's function and need for continuing care interventions. This can be done using a specific measure of function such as the FIM® (Functional Independence Measure), an international standard for the measurement of disability; using cumulative scores produces a quantitative index of the person's function. The FIM™ score has proven validity as an index of rehabilitation efficacy and can be used in acute hospitals, post-acute rehabilitation hospitalisation, nursing homes and home care.

An initial individualised care plan should be developed based on the person's overall condition and function (degree of pre- and post fracture autonomy, comorbidity, polypharmacotherapy, postfracture conditions, delirium and recovery motivation) and point in the post-hospital trajectory (intensive, extensive rehabilitation). If discharge home is planned, requests for appropriate aids can be made at this time. The education and training of patients and informal caregivers should also begin as soon as possible and continued once the patient is home.

The discharge phase: The multidisciplinary team collaborates to devise and operationalise a definitive individualised care plan for discharge. Assessment of the degree of independence and autonomy achieved by the patient during their hospital stay and recovery and their readiness for discharge can be assessed. Important arrangements for transport, follow-up, equipment and drugs should also be made by the discharge coordinator. Ultimately, verification of the patient's arrival home and that services have commenced will complete the process. If home care is being provided, care will be formally transferred to the health professional who is assigned to the patient and family, the coordinator of the rehabilitation facility or the care leader in the residential care facility.

10.3.4 Continuity of Care

Continuity of care has three aims; best quality of care, the best health outcomes for the patient and cost reduction [17], and is achieved through:

1. The transfer of information and sharing of the patient's story with other professionals
2. Timely collection of information and activation of necessary resources immediately following discharge
3. Effective discharge planning
4. Monitoring and accompaniment
5. The assessment of needs of the use and caregivers.

Continuity of care can be achieved by one health or social care professional taking responsibility for the transition between care settings and ensuring that effective care is provided throughout the transition while focusing on the person and their family [13]. Taking this responsibility ensures continuity of care from one operating unit to another and across different levels of the health and social care system. This also ensures that the complex care process is integrated and is led in a way that guarantees that the older person receives a coordinated set of interventions aimed at meeting their complex needs. This enables governance of a complex and integrated care process in its various stages and guarantees that a coordinated set of interventions aimed at satisfying complex needs is in place [18].

There are several critical issues that can lead to discharge problems:

- Lack of a planned discharge date
- A high level of support needed for family who are inadequately prepared for the discharge
- Delayed activation of community services
- Poor attention to the needs of frail older people
- Lack of intermediate care services
- Lack of residential care facilities
- Poor knowledge of formal and informal services and how to access them
- Difficulty dealing with the paperwork
- Lack of support and a sense of abandonment of caregivers [13].

10.3.5 The Nurse's Role in Discharge

Nurses have an important role in ensuring continuity of care between settings and can act as a coordinator, supporting hospital staff involved in the discharge process, reducing hospital readmissions, ensuring continuity of care and educating patients about safety in continued care [19]. Care that began in the acute hospital should be continued following discharge through specialist nurse-led care in the rehabilitation hospital, intermediate care, home care or residential care setting led by a nurse with masters' level gerontological education [9].

In many health systems, a nurse is employed as a case manager or discharge coordinator whose key role is to support discharge planning and negotiating the different parts of care services and formal and informal care networks, particularly during transfer from one service to another. This includes supporting the person who cannot directly, or through a family member, interface with the care networks themselves. The nurse case manager is responsible for [20]:

1. Care integration: ensuring coherence between what has been planned and what is achieved
2. Coordination of care: ensuring that the care plan is followed by all those involved in its provision
3. Continuity of care: ensuring the implementation of the plan of care across all areas of care.

Nurses are the most appropriate health professionals to act as case manager [21] and/or discharge coordinator because of:

- Their clinical skills
- Ability to improve the coordination of services
- They are more generalist than other professionals
- They excel in giving direct care and pay attention to the relationship between care quality and cost and the natural evolution of nursing care
- Their ability to understand the holistic needs of patients and their current and potential problems [20].

There are many skills needed by the nurse case manager including; agent of change, clinical knowledge, identification and assignment of cases, consultancy, educator, coordinator and facilitator of care, resource manager and outcome and quality manager and advocate.

10.4 Summary of Key Points for Learning

- Rehabilitation and discharge planning should begin as soon as possible after admission
- The primary outcomes of rehabilitation are independence in physical function and quality of life

- Effective rehabilitation is important in promoting independence and in enabling the patient to reach their potential and return home
- Early supported multidisciplinary rehabilitation can reduce hospital stay, improve early return to function and impact positively on both readmission rates and the level of care required
- Supported exercise and mobility include interventions involving using everyday activities as part of the rehabilitation programme to increase independence
- The discharge of an older person from an acute hospital is complex and requires careful planning and, if ineffectively conducted, can affect patient outcomes
- Nurses ensure continuity of care between settings and can act as a coordinator in the discharge process.

10.5 Recommended Further Study

- Think about a patient whose rehabilitation you are currently or were recently involved in. Based on your learning from this chapter, identify areas in their care you could improve.
- Carefully read the following article and reflect on how you might apply it to your practice: Lindberg, L. et al. (2017) Changing caring behaviours in rehabilitation after a hip fracture—A tool for empowerment? Psychology Health and Medicine 22(6):663–*672* https://doi.org/10.1080/13548506.2016.1211294.
- Examine the documentation for a patient in whose discharge you were recently involved—if possible, one for which you acted as discharge coordinator. Reflect on the quality of the discharge, bearing in mind what you have learnt from this chapter and consider how the discharge might have been improved by your actions. Identify an action plan for improving the way you approach patient discharge as a coordinator.
- Seek advice and mentorship from other expert clinicians such as physiotherapists, social workers and those who are experts in rehabilitation or discharge planning.

10.6 How to Self-Assess Learning

To identify learning achieved and the need for further study, the following strategies may be helpful:

- Examine local documentation of nursing care, regarding rehabilitation and discharge status, and use this to assess your knowledge and performance.
- Meet with specialists and other members of the team to keep up to date on new evidence and disseminate it to colleagues. The conversation in these meetings can include any recent new practices, guidance, knowledge or evidence.

References

1. British Orthopaedic Association (BOA) (2007) The care of patients with fragility fracture. British Orthopaedic Association
2. Menzies IB et al (2010) Prevention and clinical Management of hip fractures in patients with dementia. Geriatr Orthop Surg Rehabil 1(2):63–72
3. Dyer S et al (2017) Rehabilitation following hip fracture. In: Falaschi P, Marsh D (eds) Orthogeriatrics. Springer, Switzerland, pp 145–163
4. National Clinical Guideline Centre (2011) The Management of Hip Fracture in Adults. National Clinical Guideline Centre, London. www.ncgc.ac.uk
5. Olsson L-E et al (2007) Effects of nursing interventions within and integrated care pathway for patients with hip fracture. J Adv Nurs 58(2):116–125
6. Curtis L (2009) Unit costs of health & social care 2009. Personal Social Services Research Unit, Canterbury, Kent (Guideline Ref ID: CURTIS2009)
7. Sherrington C, Whitney JC, Lord SR, Herbert RD, Cumming RG, Close JC (2008) Effective exercise for the prevention of falls: a systematic review and meta-analysis. J Am Geriatr Soc 56(12):2234–2243
8. Gesar B (2017) Older patients' perception of their own capacity to regain pre-fracture function after hip fracture surgery—an explorative qualitative study. Int J Orthop Trauma Nurs 24:50–58
9. Crotty M et al (2010) Rehabilitation interventions for improving physical and psychosocial functioning after hip fracture in older people (review) 5 Copyright © 2010 The Cochrane Collaboration. Wiley
10. Maclean N, Pound P (2000) A critical review of the concept of patient motivation in the literature on physical rehabilitation. Soc Sci Med 50:495–506
11. Hitch B et al (2016) Evaluation of a team-based, transition-of-care management service on 30-day readmission rates. NC Med J 77(2):87–92
12. Gunadi S et al (2015) Development of a collaborative transitions-of-care program for heart failure patients. Am J Health Syst Pharm 72(13):1147–1152
13. Bauer M et al (2009) Hospital discharge planning for frail older people and their family. Are we delivering best practice? A review of the evidence. J Clin Nurs 18(18):2539–2546
14. Kripalani S et al (2007) Deficits in communication and information transfer between hospital-based and primary care physicians: implications for patient safety and continuity of care. JAMA 297:831
15. National Patient Safety Foundation/Institute for Healthcare Improvement (nd) Ask Me 3. http://www.npsf.org/?page=askme3
16. Blaylock A, Cason CL (1992) Discharge planning predicting patients' needs. J Gerontol Nurs 18:5–10
17. Randmaa M et al (2014) SBAR improves communication and safety climate and decreases incident reports due to communication errors in an anaesthetic clinic: a prospective intervention study. BMJ Open 4:e004268. https://doi.org/10.1136/bmjopen-2013-004268
18. Holland D, Harris M (2007) Discharge planning, transitional care, coordination of care, and continuity of care: clarifying concepts and terms from the hospital perspective. Home Health Care Serv Quart 26(4):3–19
19. Kangovi S et al (2014) The use of participatory action research to design a patient-centered community health worker care transitions intervention. Healthc (Amst) 2(2):136–144
20. Gulliford M et al (2006) What is 'continuity of care'? J Health Serv Res Policy 11(4):248–250
21. Cohen EL, Cesta TG (1993) Nursing case management: from concept to evaluation. Mosby, St Louis

11 Family Partnerships, Palliative Care and End of Life

Louise Brent, Julie Santy-Tomlinson, and Karen Hertz

The involvement of families, friends and others important to the patient has always been central in person-centred, individualised care. Following fragility fracture, many patients wish for their family and significant others to be involved in their care, both during the hospital stay and following discharge and it is often expected that families will provide, or lead, continuing care once they are discharged.

For some patients, a significant fracture such as hip fracture may be a final element of a struggle with physical and psychological decline and frailty. It may signal the nearing of, and may hasten, the end of life. For these patients, person- and family-centred care may be needed that is focused on dignity and comfort, rather than surgical intervention. More people are living longer and living with serious, life-limiting or life-threatening conditions.

Palliative care has been associated with cancer, but has evolved to include patients with a range of complex and chronic medical conditions, and focuses on conservative management and care rather than invasive medical interventions, but is not necessarily focused on the end of life, rather on comfort, symptom management, dignity and family-centred care.

In some cases, patients with fragility fractures may become seriously ill due to their frailty and the complications of the fracture or surgery. This may result in

L. Brent
National Office of Clinical Audit, St Stephen's Green, Dublin 2, Ireland

J. Santy-Tomlinson (✉)
Faculty of Biology, Medicine and Health, Division of Nursing, Midwifery and Social Work, School of Health Sciences, The University of Manchester, Manchester, UK
e-mail: Julie.santy-tomlinson@manchester.ac.uk

K. Hertz
Specialised Division, University Hospital of North Midlands, Stoke-on Trent, Staffordshire, UK
e-mail: Karen.hertz@uhnm.nhs.uk

K. Hertz, J. Santy-Tomlinson (eds.), *Fragility Fracture Nursing*, Perspectives in Nursing Management and Care for Older Adults, https://doi.org/10.1007/978-3-319-76681-2_11

sudden death but can also lead to an awareness that death is pending, but the process of dying may take several days or weeks. Patients and their families expect good end of life care that involves management of physical symptoms such as pain, breathlessness, nausea and increasing fatigue as well as the anxiety, depression and social and spiritual difficulties that can accompany the end of life. Whether the patient dies in the hospital or at home, care should be based on effective MDT working [1] that includes collaboration with the patient and their family and other informal carers.

This chapter will explore the importance of family partnerships in healthcare and approaches to palliative and end of life for care for patients with a fragility fracture.

11.1 Learning Outcomes

At the end of the chapter, the nurse will be able to:

- Discuss the role of family and friends as carers and how nurses should facilitate family involvement in care
- Discuss the concepts of palliative and end of life care following fragility fracture
- Be aware of medicolegal issues that affect decision-making in end of life care
- Define and practice effective palliative care
- Define and practice good end of life care
- Discuss the role of the fragility fracture practitioner in palliative and end of life care.

11.2 Family Partnerships and Involvement in Care

There has been significant change in the way healthcare professionals view care delivery, from a medical-centric model to a patient-centred approach. The term "patient-centred medicine" was first coined in 1969 [2], and the Picker Commonwealth Program for Patient-Centred Care (subsequently the Picker Institute) developed the term "patient-centred" in 1998 [3]. It is now acknowledged that a key priority for patients is how their own wishes and those of their families and carers are integrated throughout the care process. Healthcare workers are now expected to place an emphasis on collaborating with patients and families of all ages, at all levels of care and in all healthcare settings.

The concept of family caregiving has also developed significantly and now reflects the changing nature of "family" in society. Much informal care is given by individuals who would not traditionally be considered family members and such "informal caregiving" is recognised as an important facet of care delivery. Informal caregivers are defined as "persons without formal health care education who are caring for, or helping, a person with functional disabilities, prolonged psychiatric or physical illness, or age-related problems" [4]. Within this chapter, the term "family" will be used to encapsulate all persons who have an important relationship with the patient, e.g. relative, partner, friend and neighbour.

Families are an essential component of care, health and wellbeing; quality and safety initiatives recognise the role they play in ensuring high standards of care, and they are allies for quality and safety within the healthcare system [5]. Families often act as the primary caregivers and as advocates for patient who are not able to make decisions for themselves. They are an essential part of the patient care continuum and a fundamental characteristic of holistic care is that nurses must collaborate with others to achieve best practice [6].

There are four keys factors to be considered in relation to patient and family involvement: dignity and respect, information sharing, participation and collaboration. When a patient is admitted to a hospital or other healthcare setting, the reason for admission is often the focus; but, to be holistic, practitioners need to consider a myriad of factors. The reason the patient requires care may not be their own most significant concern. When asked, patients will tell healthcare staff what is worrying them most and it is up to practitioners to really listen and respect their wishes. Nurses spend the most time with the patient and therefore have a central role to play in relaying and advocating for the patient's and family's wishes and concerns, taking into consideration their knowledge, values, beliefs and cultural norms.

Communication is a key ingredient for ensuring timely and appropriate information sharing between healthcare staff and the patient and family. It is known that: "…no matter how knowledgeable a clinician might be, if he or she is not able to open good communication with the patient, he or she may be of no help" [7]; good communication also impacts on patient outcomes and healthcare staff experience. Patients' perceptions of the quality of the healthcare they receive are highly dependent on the quality of their interactions and communication with clinicians and team members [8]. All information shared should be unbiased and relevant; asking the patient or family what it is they need to know or better understand can help avoid frustrations, miscommunication, upset and worry. Practitioners must also communicate the same message to the patient and family to avoid misunderstandings and ensure that they are able to make the most appropriate decision about their care. This two-way dialogue encourages collaboration in achieving good quality decision-making and a better ultimate experience for all involved. Practitioners need to adopt a culture of collaboration with families and patients and have a clear programme and structure to ensure this happens at every level of the organisation.

11.2.1 Assessment

In the first instance, a comprehensive holistic understanding of the family's role in the care of the patient needs to be achieved and documented. Principal issues for consideration include:

- Who is the legal "next of kin"?
- Do the family want to provide care?

- Who, if anyone, has previously provided care and what was the care?
- How often is this care required?
- Is it enough to meet the needs of the patient/family?
- Is the environment in which care is provided suitable and adequate?
- What resources or equipment does the patient require, i.e. walking aids?
- What kind of formal care is in place? How often does the patient see their doctor, public health nurse or other carers?
- How have they been managing?
- Have they any worries or perceptions that need to be discussed?
- Are there financial worries for the patient or family in relation to the care required and being provided?
- Is this responsibility causing undue distress?

Families have other priorities such as work and other dependents such as children that need to be considered, and healthcare staff should never assume that the family wish or are able to give care, nor should judgements be made if they prefer not to be involved in direct care. It is important to establish how much support has been, and can be, given by non-family members, the costs associated and how effective this is. Family should be asked if they are aware of any voluntary or community-based support that can provide resources. Grants and financial help may be available that patients and family can access from social care agencies or voluntary organisations.

The involvement of families in care after discharge requires careful planning and organisation during the discharge planning process, beginning with an open conversation with the patient and their family to ensure that everyone understands what the implications of decisions are. Arrangements should be made for equipment and facilities in the home. Families may need to develop specific care skills, and arrangements need to be in place for this so that they understand issues such as patient limitations and potential continuing progress towards recovery. Should a decision be made that the patient will be discharged permanently or temporarily to residential care, the implications for the family such as social and financial aspects need to be carefully considered with the help of social work practitioners.

11.2.2 Caregiver Burden

Voluntary or informal caregiving is a choice and should not be an expectation. Practitioners must take account of the likelihood of caregiver burden, defined as "the physical, emotional and financial responses of a caregiver to the changes and demands caused by providing help to another person with a physical or mental disability" [9]. This is commonly exhibited by families and carers of patients with long-term chronic diseases or acute prolonged episodes of care that can impact physically, psychologically and socially on carers' health and quality of life and, therefore, on the quality of care provided.

Common features of caregiver burden include tiredness, emotional distress, conflicts, financial difficulties, not meeting the care needs of the patient and changes in the relationship between the patient and carer. A significant cause of these problems is lack of preparation for the caregiver role, poor communication, lack of understanding and appropriate training for the carer, lack of support or perceived support and poor awareness of how to access resources or to navigate health and social care systems.

There is a relationship between informal caregiver wellbeing and the physical and psychological health of the patient, so health and social care services need to ensure that carers are fully supported [10]. This can only be achieved with continued contact and communication. Regular reviews of the care requirements should take place that will enable the carer to be supported. There is a limit to what is reasonable and achievable through informal care and longer-term plans may need to be put in place if care needs are prolonged or carers are not able to cope due to care burden.

11.2.3 Legal and Ethical Considerations

The patient is the key decision-maker in their care but, if a patient does not possess the capacity to make decisions about their care, practitioners must act in their best interests to determine who is the correct and legal person to make and inform any decisions made. To do this, the practitioner must understand the terms capacity, advanced healthcare directive (AHD) or living will and co-decision-maker.

Capacity is defined as the person's ability to understand, at the time that a decision is to be made, the nature and consequences of the decision to be made by him or her in the context of the available choices at that time [11]. An expression by a person of his or her will and preferences concerning treatment decisions that may arise if the person subsequently lacks the capacity to make such decisions is known as a living will or an advanced healthcare directive (AHD). The person may appoint someone (known as a co-decision-maker) to jointly or solely make decisions, through a legal, witnessed and documented process, on their behalf should they not possess the capacity to do so.

11.3 Palliative and End of Life Care

For some patients, their fragility fracture, especially a hip fracture, may be an event that will hasten the end of life. Some patients, especially those who are already frail, may be unable to survive the physiological stress of the fracture and subsequent surgery. At these times, the principles of palliative care should be applied. The World Health Organization [12] defines palliative care as; "an approach that improves the quality of life of patients and their families facing the problems associated with life-threatening illness, through the prevention and relief of suffering by means of early identification and impeccable assessment and treatment of pain and other problems, physical, psychosocial and spiritual". The fundamental aims of palliative care include [12]:

- Providing adequate pain relief and minimising discomfort by providing symptom relief
- Affirming life and regarding dying as a normal process
- Intending neither to hasten nor postpone death
- Integrating the psychological and spiritual aspects of patient care
- Offering a support system to help patients live as actively as possible until death
- Offering to provide a system of support to help the family cope during the patient's illness and death and in their own bereavement
- Working collaboratively as a team to address the needs of patients and their families, including bereavement counselling, if indicated
- Enhancing quality of life and positively influencing the course of illness
- Applicable early in the course of illness, in conjunction with other therapies that are intended to prolong life, such as chemotherapy or radiation therapy, and includes those investigations needed to better understand and manage distressing clinical complications.

It is important to note that surgery for hip fracture may remain the most effective way to manage pain for patients who are reaching the end of life, so the reasons for the decision to undertake surgery must be clearly explained to the patient and family and ethical decision-making employed as discussed earlier.

Palliative care is not limited by time and care should be delivered based on needs as they arise. It can take place in primary care, in acute hospitals and in long-term and hospice care facilities. More people are living longer with more co-morbidities and, unfortunately, the insult of a major fracture such as a hip fracture can see the patient's health decline and ultimately result in end of life. It is estimated that there were approximately 54.6 million deaths worldwide in 2011 and that 9% of those were due to injuries [13]. Men have a higher risk of mortality after a hip fracture, but women are also at substantial risk of death; this risk exceeds the lifetime risk of death from breast cancer, uterine cancer and ovarian cancer combined. Many patients who survive a hip fracture do not regain their pre-fracture functional level, and almost one third lose their independence [14]. Practitioners must be equipped for, and expect to deliver, end of life and palliative care in the orthopaedic and orthogeriatric setting routinely rather than as an exception.

When considering the philosophy of "end of life care", Dame Cicely Saunders said: "You matter because you are you, and you matter to the end of your life. We will do all we can not only to help you die peacefully, but also to live until you die". Her words reflect the human responsibility to care for others in a humanistic and compassionate way until the end of their life.

There are many responsibilities in end of life care, ranging from communicating with individuals and families about their care and preferences; to observing, discussing and recording any changes in condition and offering compassion and support. A broad range of care skills are needed along with awareness of the values which underpin this philosophy of care. When providing end of life care, practitioners should [15]:

- Treat people compassionately
- Listen to people
- Communicate clearly and sensitively
- Identify and meet the communication needs of each individual
- Acknowledge pain and distress and take action
- Recognise when someone may be entering the last few days and hours of life
- Involve people in decisions about their care and respect their wishes
- Keep the person who is reaching the end of their life and those important to them up to date with any changes in condition
- Document a summary of conversations and decisions
- Seek further advice if needed
- Look after yourself and your colleagues and seek support if you need it.

End of life and palliative care are not limited to the acute hospital and can be provided in a range of settings including the community, care homes and hospices. Practitioners need to be attuned to noticing when a person is nearing the end of life or actively dying. How the patient and family are communicated with during this phase of life will depend on the individual patient. As much as possible, this should be patient-led and the nurse should proceed with gentle, honest answers, using a language the person understands. If the patient is uncomfortable, or does not wish to talk about death, it is important to respect their wishes. It is crucial, however, to have sensitive conversations with families and carers to prepare them for impending death.

Good nursing care for those at the end of their life should include physical, emotional and psychological aspects of care along with spiritual support. The process of dying creates multiple emotions and feelings for all involved; the patient, family, carers and the care providers. It can be very stressful and complex. It is helpful to use tools to assist in identifying indicators that someone is approaching their end of life such as the Gold Standards Framework (GSF) [16] and the Palliative Performance Scale 2 (PPS). Nurses play a key role in helping the patient throughout this natural process. The gentle "winding down" at the very end of life can be very peaceful as the body starts to let go, so if the patient is distressed or restless, this can be disrupted.

11.4 Summary of Main Points for Learning

- A patient's family and other people meaningful to them are important participants in the care process and need to be recognised as such. Good communication and collaboration with families can be central to achieving high-quality care and good patient outcomes.

- Much care is provided by family members and other informal carers following discharge. Informal carers need to be educated and supported by practitioners during the discharge planning process to enable them to provide effective care. Potential carer burden must be recognised and support must be provided to prevent it. Informal care cannot continue limitlessly and other more permanent formal care may need to be arranged.
- Fragility fracture, particularly hip fracture, may be a signal of, or hasten, the end of life. Palliative and end of life care are, therefore, important aspects of the care process in both hospital and community settings. Physical, psychological, emotional and spiritual care need to be provided in a sensitive and compassionate manner.

11.5 Suggested Further Study

- Find local and national guidance for palliative and end of life care, and use these to identify ways in which care might be improved with respect to these aspects of care.

11.6 How to Self-Assess Learning

To identify learning achieved and the need for further study, the following strategies may be helpful:

- Seek feedback from families and carers about their perceptions of the collaborative, family-centred approach employed in your unit.
- Seek advice and mentorship from experts in end of life and palliative care.
- Undertake written reflection about your experiences of end of life and palliative care, and consider whether care could be improved.
- Peer review by colleagues can be used to assess individual progress and practice but should not be too formal. There should be open discussion within the team. Weekly case conferences can identify nurse-focused issues and enable the exchange of expertise. Expertise is conveyed to the various members of the MDT by educational initiatives and by fostering a culture where all the patients' problems are considered.

References

1. NICE (2011) End of life care for adults: quality standard 13. National Institute for Health and Care Excellence. https://www.nice.org.uk/guidance/qs13
2. Balint M et al (1969) Training medical students in patient-centered medicine. Compr Psychiatry 10(4):249–258

3. Shaller D (2007) Patient-centred care: what does it take? Picker Institute and the Commonwealth Fund. http://cgp.pickerinstitute.org/wp-content/uploads/2010/12/shaller.pdf
4. Lethin C et al (2016) Formal support for informal caregivers to older persons with dementia through the course of the disease: an exploratory, cross-sectional study. BMC Geriatr 16:32
5. Bezold C (2004) The future of patient-centred care: scenarios, visions, and audacious goals. J Altern Complement Med 11(s1):s77–s84
6. Hall C, Ritchie D (2013) What is nursing? Exploring theory and practice, 3rd edn. Sage/Learning Matters, London
7. Institute for Healthcare Communication (2011) Impact of communication in healthcare. http://healthcarecomm.org/about-us/impact-of-communication-in-healthcare/
8. Wanzer MB et al (2004) Perceptions of health care providers' communication: relationships between patient-centred communication and satisfaction. Health Commun 16(3):363–384
9. Pearlin LI et al (1990) Caregiving and the stress process; an overview of concepts and their measures. Gerontologist 30:583–594
10. Falaschi P, Eleuteri S (2017) The psychological health of patients and their caregivers. In: Falaschi P, Marsh D (eds) Orthogeriatrics. Switzerland, Springer, pp 201–211
11. Office of the Attorney General. Assisted Decision-Making (Capacity) Act 2015. http://www.irishstatutebook.ie/eli/2015/act/64/enacted/en/html
12. World Health Organization (2014) Global atlas of palliative care at the end of life. www.who.int/nmh/Global_Atlas_of_Palliative_Care.pdf
13. World Health Organization (2013) Global health estimates. Causes of death 2000–2011. www.who.int/healthinfo/global_burden_disease/en
14. Kates SL, Mears SC (2011) A guide to improving the care of patients with fragility fractures. Geriatr Orthop Surg Rehabil 2(1):5–37
15. Royal College of Nursing (2015) RCN end of life care- roles and responsibilities. http://rcnendoflife.org.uk/my-role/
16. Royal College of General Practitioners (2016) The Gold Standards Framework Proactive Identification Guidance (PIG). https://www.goldstandardsframework.org.uk/cd-content/uploads/files/PIG/NEW%20PIG%20-%20%20%2020.1.17%20KT%20vs17.pdf

Orthogeriatric Nursing

12

Julie Santy-Tomlinson, Karen Hertz, and Magdalena Kaminska

Nursing is central to good care for the patient with a fragility fracture and makes a major contribution to positive outcomes. Nurses are the largest group of health professionals in the orthogeriatric team and they are the one group who are present for the full 24-hour span during hospitalisation. They are also most likely to work across organisational boundaries, acting as links between the patient's home and local community, the hospital, the outpatient/ambulatory setting and other organisations.

Nurses who work in the orthogeriatric setting must be able to clearly articulate their role and value so that they can inform patients, their families and other members of the MDT what to expect from them. No single healthcare profession can provide care to fragility fracture patients in isolation, but it is known that patients' outcomes are improved if there is full collaboration across all disciplines making up the "orthogeriatric" team [1] and patients with a fragility fracture have numerous complex care needs that need a team approach that includes skilled, compassionate nursing. Although this chapter is concerned with orthogeriatric nursing generally, it is impossible to ignore the fact that of all fragility fractures, hip fracture is the most significant injury: it is the most common reason for admission to an orthopaedic ward, accounts for much orthopaedic bed occupancy and is a large portion of the

J. Santy-Tomlinson (✉)
Faculty of Biology, Medicine and Health, Division of Nursing, Midwifery and Social Work, School of Health Sciences, The University of Manchester, Manchester, UK
e-mail: Julie.santy-tomlinson@manchester.ac.uk

K. Hertz
Specialised Division, University Hospital of North Midlands, Stoke-on Trent, Staffordshire, UK
e-mail: Karen.hertz@uhnm.nhs.uk

M. Kaminska
Faculty of Health Sciences, Department of Primary Health Care, Pomeranian Medical University, Szczecin, Poland

K. Hertz, J. Santy-Tomlinson (eds.), *Fragility Fracture Nursing*, Perspectives in Nursing Management and Care for Older Adults, https://doi.org/10.1007/978-3-319-76681-2_12

total cost of all fragility fractures. It is also the most expensive fracture in terms of volume and unit costs. Complexity of patient needs, prevalence, number of bed days and cost means that the focus of inpatient care tends to relate predominantly to this category of injury. However, the principal skills and knowledge needed to look after hip fracture patients well must be applied across the management of all older patients with fractures and include all fundamental aspects of nursing care for the adult as well as highly specialised interventions for older people.

The aim of this chapter is to consider the nature of orthogeriatric nursing and to explore its theoretical, political and professional aspects.

12.1 Learning Outcomes

At the end of the chapter, and following further study, the nurse will be able to:

- Explain the nature of orthogeriatric nursing, using adult and geriatric nursing theory and philosophy
- Explore the professional, ethical, legal and political aspects of orthogeriatric nursing
- Articulate the value of orthogeriatric nursing in achieving good outcomes for patients
- Discuss the importance of skill, knowledge and education in providing effective care to patients with fragility fractures.

12.2 Nursing

Nursing is broad and complex, so defining nursing enables nurses to explain to patients, families and others what they can expect from them. The ICN [2] defines both "nursing" and "a nurse" (see Box 12.1) to highlight the expanse of the nursing role across the entire lifespan, in all communities and with people with all healthcare needs. These definitions help to illuminate some of the central aspects of nursing care

Box 12.1: International Council of Nurses (ICN) Definitions of Nursing and a Nurse [1]

Definition of Nursing (Short Version)

"Nursing encompasses autonomous and collaborative care of individuals of all ages, families, groups and communities, sick or well and in all settings. Nursing includes the promotion of health, prevention of illness, and the care of ill, disabled and dying people. Advocacy, promotion of a safe environment, research, participation in shaping health policy and in patient and health systems management, and education are also key nursing roles".

Definition of a Nurse

"The nurse is a person who has completed a program of basic, generalized nursing education and is authorized by the appropriate regulatory authority to practice nursing in his/her country. Basic nursing education is a formally recognized program of study providing a broad and sound foundation in the behavioral, life, and nursing sciences for the general practice of nursing, for a leadership role, and for post-basic education for specialty or advanced nursing practice. The nurse is prepared and authorized (1) to engage in the general scope of nursing practice, including the promotion of health, prevention of illness, and care of physically ill, mentally ill, and disabled people of all ages and in all health care and other community settings; (2) to carry out health care teaching; (3) to participate fully as a member of the health care team; (4) to supervise and train nursing and health care auxiliaries; and (5) to be involved in research".

that include activities related to the scope of nursing; how care is given; what knowledge, skills and education are needed and how nursing constitutes a profession.

Nursing is both a caring art and a science and it encompasses a distinct body of knowledge, separate from that of medical or allied health professional colleagues. Knowledge is specific information about something and caring is behaviour that demonstrates compassion and respect for another, but these simplified concepts do not truly reflect the synthesis of both knowledge and the art of caring that makes orthogeriatric nursing unique [3].

12.3 The Orthogeriatric Patient

Patients with fragility fractures present across the spectrum of health service providers including general practice, community services, acute care services including emergency portals, operating departments, inpatient and outpatient services and hospital- or community-based rehabilitation services. Care takes place in an environment that is largely not conducive to the care of frail older people. The provision of safe, effective care for hospitalised patients following hip fracture is particularly complex and demands a focus on achieving best outcomes for frail elderly hospitalised patients. This complexity is generated by multiple interlocking problems related to both breadth (range) and depth (severity) of healthcare need [4] related to three main characteristics; the person, the fracture and the care environment—all of which have a significant impact on patient care outcomes [5]. Orthogeriatric patients have usually fallen, often have multiple co-morbidities and are frequently frail. These problems interact in the aftermath of fragility fracture to increase care needs because of the increased physiological demands of the pre-, peri- and post-operative recovery and rehabilitation phases of care.

12.4 Care Quality

Nursing is underpinned by a set of core personal and professional values, and the meaning of "quality care" varies depending on whether it is viewed from the perspective of the care giver or the care receiver but tends to be based on six core elements: a holistic approach, patient empowerment, professional accountability, patient safety, integrated teamwork and efficiency and effectiveness [6].

Compassion is a quality that enables nurses to be motivated to provide effective, person-centred care and is essential to quality nursing care; it includes empathy, respect and dignity, qualities that require understanding and recognition of another's suffering and a desire to do something about it. It is these qualities that enable nurses to see every patient as an individual and to humanise their care [7]. This is always important, but particularly when those receiving care are vulnerable as in the case of an elderly frail person who has suffered a hip fracture.

Quality care is significantly affected by communication, but even basic communication with vulnerable older adults accessing healthcare services is complex. Problems between individuals, families, caregivers and health professionals usually occur simply because communication is not effective. Everyone is a unique individual with personal values, beliefs, perceptions, culture and understanding of how the world operates. Fragility fractures predominantly, but not exclusively, affect older adults, who formed their opinions, values and beliefs in a very different society to that of the younger people who provide their care, and there can be a cultural age gap that leads to misunderstanding. Nurses need to understand the world from the perspective of an older person to communicate with them effectively and the sensory impairments and potential cognitive dysfunction that are common in older people add to the complexity of developing therapeutic communication. Understanding the acute needs of a patient with a fragility fracture and its management, as well as the chronic underlying diagnosis of osteoporosis and its treatment and impact, add to the already considerable complexity of being an older person with a set of co-morbid medical conditions and social and psychological intricacies resulting from primary and secondary ageing. Effective communication is two-way and involves ensuring that the messages are understood. Barriers to communication may need to be removed in simple ways such as ensuring glasses, hearing aids, interpreters and visual graphics are used to aid communication along with involvement of family friends, caregivers or advocates who know the patient best.

The success of healthcare delivery is often examined by measuring health status, outcomes, readmission rates, length of stay, complication rates and mortality [8], but these do not necessarily capture the specific contribution of nursing. Length of stay is a misleading measure for success as there are decreased levels of expert nursing care when patients are discharged or transferred too early [9]. Appropriate indicators of the quality of nursing care could include measures such as patient comfort and quality of life, safety outcomes (including healthcare-associated infection, pressure ulcers, falls and drug administration errors) and patient satisfaction [8]. In orthogeriatric care, nurse-sensitive indicators might be developed for; pain, delirium, pressure ulcers/injuries, hydration and nutrition, constipation, prevention of secondary infections and venous thromboembolism (VTE) [5].

12.5 The Unique Contribution of Nursing to Orthogeriatric Patient Outcomes

Nursing care priorities are the fundamental aspects of nursing care including; comfort, hygiene, pain management, nutrition, hydration, remobilisation and rehabilitation. Evidenced-based nursing can coexist with medical models of care, reducing the risk of developing complications, aiming to reduce the risk of morbidity and mortality, whilst improving recovery, maintaining functional ability and improving patient outcomes and experiences [5].

Nurses often become specialists in specific aspects of healthcare to enable them to focus on providing skilled care based on up-to-date knowledge to a defined group, so they often work in teams with other specialists such as medical practitioners and therapists, collaborating in pathways and sharing evidence across professions. Orthogeriatrics was first used to describe collaboration between the specialties of orthopaedic surgery and geriatric medicine but has come to denote a multidisciplinary approach to the hospital care of patients with fragility fractures that recognises the complex specific needs of this group. The concept of orthogeriatrics recognises the need to understand the holistic healthcare needs of frail, elderly patients with multiple health problems at the same time as working towards the best outcomes following fragility fracture [10].

12.6 Health Improvement and Health Promotion

The education of patients for health improvement is often the role of nurses because they are the largest group of healthcare providers, but their actual and potential contribution to the management of chronic disease is underappreciated. The reasons for the prevalence of chronic disease in communities are complex; although there is an enormous body of evidence confirming how it can be avoided and treated, prevalence continues to rise and outcomes remain poor. Many patients are often inadequately informed, do not take responsibility for their condition and do not comply with instructions. Management of osteoporosis as a chronic condition provides an example of this; it is difficult to manage as it is often silent and the treatment can be unpalatable; concordance with oral bisphosphonates is poor, particularly in those patients not managed by ongoing nurse coordinator intervention. Nurses working in all settings play a central role in educating and coaching patients and families towards behaviour change that can positively influence health and healthcare outcomes following fragility fracture. The success of health improvement initiatives is reliant on nurses building trust with patients and families and working with them towards improvements in bone health and other related health domains. Every fall and fracture is an opportunity to prevent the next fall or fracture by MDT collaboration to prevent further falls and manage osteoporosis [11]. Nurses must be empowered to use the time they spend giving care with patients and families to educate them about the cause of fragility fractures and involve patients in developing an individualised plan of care for bone health.

12.7 The Nursing Resource

Providing high-quality nursing care is labour intensive and requires an educated and highly skilled workforce led by experienced leaders of care who can direct a team of nurses who are qualified to plan evidence-based care and manage its delivery alongside well-trained and supervised support workers. Because of an ageing workforce and lack of political will to adequately fund nursing, global availability of enough skilled nurses to provide this fundamental and advanced care is a constant source of concern. It has, however, been demonstrated that an increase in a nurses' workload by one patient, from eight to nine patients per qualified nurse, increases the likelihood of an inpatient dying within 30 days of admission by 7% [12], indicating "missed care" [13] because of difficulties for nurses in undertaking actions to prevent complications and subsequent death.

12.8 Education for Orthogeriatric Care

Competence is a hallmark of professional practice [14] but cannot be achieved if nurses do not have the requisite knowledge and skills to deliver care effectively to specific groups of patients. The benefits of providing highly skilled and specialist nursing of fragility fracture patients by practitioners with advanced, specific education have not been explored, but the development of specialist orthogeriatric nursing education could have a positive impact on patient outcomes [9]. Orthogeriatric nursing is an emerging and highly specialised branch of adult nursing that requires skills in both the care of the older person and the care of the orthopaedic and trauma patient so that the practitioner can bring both sets of skills together and use them to provide expert care to patients following fragility fracture with complex care needs that cannot be met without a deep understanding of how both age and frailty, as well as skeletal fragility and injury, impact on the planning and implementation of care. This requires specialist practice that applies knowledge and skills brought together from both nursing disciplines and knowledge and skills from partner professional specialities. Unfortunately, nurses are not well prepared to look after orthogeriatric patients as they have usually worked in orthopaedic trauma units and been educated for the care of adults with musculoskeletal problems rather than specifically to work with frail older people with complex needs. This can lead to the more complex needs of older people not being met. There is, consequently, an important education and skills gap and, at present, there are limited education resources available to support professional development of specialist orthogeriatric nurses.

12.9 Summary of Main Points for Learning

The global shortage of nurses is now chronic and, unless the nursing resource is protected and grows, the potential of nursing to impact on patient outcomes and quality of fragility fracture care for patients with fragility fractures will be unmet [9].

"Looking after hip fracture patients well is a lot cheaper than looking after them badly" [15] and without a significant nursing resource to do the "looking after well", care will never be cost effective, and chronic health problems will never be prevented. Nurses are central to the coordination, provision and monitoring of orthogeriatric care.

12.10 Suggested Further Study

Write a written reflection on how your learning from this chapter, and the entire book, reflects your current practice.

12.11 How to Self-Assess Learning

Share your thoughts about the reflection you have written with your manager, mentor or preceptor and identify the ways in which you can become a more effective orthogeriatric practitioner.

References

1. Hall C, Ritchie D (2013) What is nursing? Exploring theory and practice, 3rd edn. Sage/Learning Matters, London
2. International Council of Nurses (ICN) (2002) Definition of nursing. http://www.icn.ch/who-we-are/icn-definition-of-nursing/
3. Cipriano P (2007) Celebrating the art and science of nursing. Am Nurse Today 2(5):8
4. Rankin J, Regan S (2004) Complex needs: the future of social care. Institute for public policy research/Turning Point. http://www.ippr.org/files/images/media/files/publication/2011/05/Meeting_Complex_Needs_full_1301.pdf?noredirect=1
5. Hertz K, Santy-Tomlinson J (2017) The nursing role. In: Falaschi P, Marsh D (eds) Orthogeriatrics. Springer, Cham, pp 131–144
6. McSherry R (2012) Quality of nursing care. In: McSherry W, McSherry R, Watson R (eds) Care in nursing: principles values and skills. Oxford University Press, Oxford
7. Baillie L, Black S (2015) Professional values in nursing. CRC, London
8. Maben J et al (2012) High quality care metrics for nursing. National Nursing Research Unit, King's College London. http://eprints.soton.ac.uk/346019/1/High-Quality-Care-Metrics-for-Nursing----Nov-2012.pdf
9. Brent L et al (2018) Nursing care of fragility fracture patients. Injury needs completing when published online (in press)
10. Falaschi P, Marsh D (2017) Orthogeriatrics. Springer, Cham
11. Martin FC (2017) Frailty, sarcopenia, falls and fractures. In: Falaschi P, Marsh D (eds) Orthogeriatrics. Springer, Cham, pp 47–62
12. Aiken L et al (2014) Nurse staffing and education and hospital mortality in nine European countries: a retrospective observational study. Lancet 383(993):1824–1830
13. Recio-Saucedo A et al (2017) What impact does nursing care left undone have on patient outcomes? Review of the literature. J Clin Nurs. https://doi.org/10.1111/jocn.140589
14. Drozd M et al (2007) The inherent components of the orthopaedic nursing role: an exploratory study. J Orthop Nurs 11(1):43–52
15. Sahota O, Currie C (2008) Hip fracture care: all change. Editorial. Age Ageing 37:128–129

Index

K. Hertz, J. Santy-Tomlinson (eds.), *Fragility Fracture Nursing*, Perspectives in Nursing Management and Care for Older Adults, https://doi.org/10.1007/978-3-319-76681-2

www.ingramcontent.com/pod-product-compliance
Lightning Source LLC
LaVergne TN
LVHW082235200926
848484LV00008B/2359
* 9 7 8 1 0 1 3 2 7 3 7 1 1 *